LIFE FORCE

The Miraculous Power of

Qi Gong

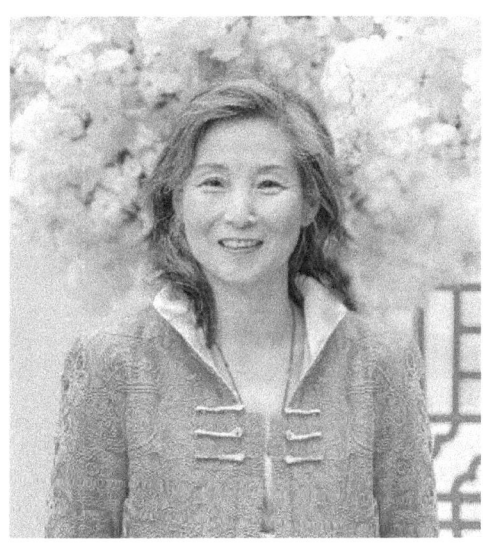

By Master Teresa W. Y. Yeung

DISCLAIMER

This book may not be resold. No part of it can be reproduced in any form by means of electronic or mechanical, including: photocopying, recording or by any information storage and retrieval system without written permission from Teresa Yeung (Master Teresa®).

This publication contains the opinions and ideas of its author, practitioners of Qi Gong and associates. It is intended to provide helpful and informative material on the subjects addressed in the publication. It is sold with the understanding that the author, the publisher or its associates are not engaged in rendering medical, health or any other kind of personal professional services in the book. The reader should consult his or her medical, health, or other competent professional before adopting any of the suggestions in the book or drawing inferences from it.

The author, publisher and its associates specifically disclaim all responsibility for any liability, loss or risk, personal or otherwise, which is incurred as a consequence, directly or indirectly of the use or application of any of the contents of this book.

CONTENTS

I WOULD LIKE TO THANK

My family, friends and students for supporting my journey and contributing to this book with your testaments to the miraculous power of Qi Gong

Rebecca, **Jacqueline** and **Daniel,** for being my wonderful children and practicing Qi Gong with me, and being a part of my path for many years

Dave Watson for helping me to strategize and support in my path with all the channeling readings

Sherree Felstead for showing me how to put a book together and sharing my life experience in writing

Master Wu, for guiding me on this path in which I can be of service to humanity by empowering people with the gift of self-healing.

Do You Believe Qi Gong (Chi Gong) Can Work for You?

In her first book: *"Life Force: The Miraculous Power of Qi Gong"*, Master Teresa Yeung wants to bring the message that Qi Gong is for the 21st century. When you change your energy, you change your life.

It is a book of encouragement and she wishes to motivate you to do more about your life by reading the inspirational life-changing success stories of herself, her family, friends, students and practitioners of Qi Gong. She wants to give you "hope" and direction by sharing how others have created their own miracles.

Her Wu's Health & Fitness Qi Gong™ - mentioned in this book - is a distilled essence of her Qi Gong, proven successful and includes the best of the masters over thousands of years. It is simple to do and almost effortless in 8 steps, and can change your energy quickly and easily. It reduces anxiety, stress and frustrations. It is good for all ages to do.

Life Force is also like a reference book and answers many commonly asked questions about energy work. Master Yeung wants to ensure readers that practicing Qi Gong is not a waste of time and it has tremendous benefits. It also illustrates the connection between the different "knots" of energy so that practitioners will be able to understand how vital Qi (life force) is for a healthy body. There are many examples of energy work covered in the book.

One way of using the book is to read a page or two per day for the next few months while practicing Qi Gong. Not only will it be a motivator, but also help practitioners build and sustain a life-long self-practice. An ongoing Qi Gong practice can achieve miraculous results.

If you are looking for a book on Qi Gong forms only, Master Teresa's videos, online programs are available and easy to follow.

Master Teresa's main message is empowerment:

You can do it.

You have hope.

Change your thought.

Never give up on yourself.

Be your own healer.

FOREWORD

By Dr. Lynda Mainwaring, PhD C. Psychology, University of Toronto
(Toronto, Canada)

Today, more than ever, we need ways to help us relax, de-stress, learn efficiently, and keep us calm and composed as we navigate the often frantic paces of modern life. Practicing Qi Gong can do this. Qi Gong is an ancient Chinese form of meditation that helps to create an internal place of solace and healing. The term is not easily translated but has been construed as "life energy", life force", and "vital energy". It is a stress reduction and meditative technique that uses breath, movement, energy management, and inner guidance to help individuals create healthy internal personal environments. Recent scientific evidence has shown that the practice of Qi Gong, like other mindfulness-based stress reduction techniques, changes brain structures and activates the parasympathetic nervous system.

I first met Master Teresa® at the University of Toronto after teaching my four-year Health Psychology class. I learned how useful the practice of Qi Gong was for quieting the body and the mind and creating an inner calm. Often, I raced to Master Teresa's class after work and it was not until half way through the class that I could feel the stress of the day's activities dissipating. I became aware of just how stressed I was, how my mind and body systems were racing, and how Qi Gong could facilitate a peaceful state of inner calm and relaxation. After class students shared how they, too, felt relaxed and calm with a heightened sense of self and the present moment.

The practice of Qi Gong as a stress reduction tool or a mind centering tool is something that everyone can learn and do. Daily practice can heighten one's sense of wellbeing. As a psychologist, I am keenly aware of how important it is to be able to manage oneself, to control and regulate emotions, to dissipate the impact of daily stresses, to take time to be in the present moment, to enjoy the richness of the simple natural things in life, and to enhance physical and psychological well-being. Qi Gong can help people do all these things.

   Learning Qi Gong from Master Teresa Yeung is a carefully guided journey into greater health and understanding of one's self. The gift of carrying on the tradition from her mentor, Master Wu, was bestowed upon her and she builds on his teachings with passion, clarity and insight. Master Teresa® shares her wisdom with her students generously so others may learn and benefit from this ancient form. She treats each individual with great care and compassion. This book has been compiled with sincere expressions of what Qi Gong has done or can do for people.

   Individuals from different walks of life have been brought together by Master Teresa® to share their experiences and benefits of Qi Gong. I hope their stories inspire you to enhance your practice or begin to learn how to use Qi Gong to enrich your wellbeing and journey through life. The mind and body are powerful; they are ours to care for and develop the best we can.
I hope you enjoy your journey with Master Teresa® on the path to where you want to be.

Dr. Lynda Mainwaring, PhD

1. THE ORIGINS OF QI GONG

In the beginning, it was believed that some people copied and imitated the movements of animals to become the movements of Qi Gong and Kung Fu. The Chinese language is tonal without syllables and the official language is Mandarin; however, there are many other dialects (regional languages), depending on where the people are residing. Each syllable has a number of different meanings, depending on how it is pronounced. Mandarin has four tones; Cantonese has between six to nine tones and Taiwanese has seven tones.

Qi, Chi or Ki

Chi, Ki or **Qi** pronounced as "chee", means "life force energy". In Mandarin, it is translated as Qi. The Cantonese way is Chi and the Japanese way is Ki. When it is written in traditional Chinese it is 氣, in simplified Chinese it is 气 and Japanese 気.
***Traditional Chinese is used in Hong Kong and Taiwan, and simplified Chinese has been used in the People's Republic of China since 1956.**

Throughout this book I will be using the Qi spelling.

Chinese Qi Gong, Chi Gong or Ki Gong or Chi Kung

In ancient times, the days of Emperors, Qi Gong was used to serve the Royal Family. After 1949, Qi Gong was better mastered by the general public and has been used as a preventative and self-healing method. In China, Qi Gong is being taught in medical colleges and research centers. Doctors need to learn Qi Gong. Large hospitals have Qi Gong research departments conducting clinical research, and in some of them, patients can request Qi Gong healing treatments (external Qi transmission) across China.

Qi Gong exercises are defined as using movements, visualization, breathing and mind control. The person practicing performs an interchange of universal energy with his or her own internal energy to make a new kind of energy or Qi. Qi Gong can have movements or no movements. There are hundreds of different kinds of Qi Gong. To understand more about Qi Gong, you can visit: http://www.wikipedia.org.

Blessings of Ascended Masters

In Chinese culture, there is only one master in each family of discipline, and each famous mountain has one family of discipline. One example is Kung Fu, which consists of boxing, weaponry and Qi Gong.

Different teachings create different energy. Masters pass on their knowledge with their Qi (Chi) to students, and to the next master together with their blessings. Worshiping ancestors or visiting the graveyard on memorial days carry similar meaning – asking for family blessings. It is believed that the master of the family carries the blessings of the teachings and Qi of their ascended masters.

When I was learning Qi Gong, my master sent his Qi to me. He said that: "Receiving Qi from me is the fastest way to jumpstart your Qi".

The Qi of a master is developed by learning, practicing and training their Qi, and also receiving Qi from their teachers. Teachers teach students, students become teachers. Improved Qi carries a certain healing vibration and is passed on from generation to generation. Learned, practiced and trained by a good teacher is therefore important in the growth of our Qi.

Neigong, Waigong, Wushu, Kung Fu and Qi Gong

There are many Chinese terms relating to cultivating Qi, which is confusing to many non-Chinese students. For example, there are phrases like "neigong 內功"and "waigong 外功". Many interpret these phrases to say "neigong" energy or "waigong" energy. Students will come to me, asking what method cultivates neigong or waigong energy. This question usually shows confusion for those who are not Chinese. For Chinese people it's poetic, because we like to use simple, classic words to describe complex meanings.

A discipline, method or exercise is called "Gong". "Nei" means inside or inner and "wai" is defined as outside or external. For example, when you do Kung Fu - which is like boxing - you are primarily focused on moving your arms and legs. Your arms, legs, hands, feet are all external parts of the body and you are looking outside. That is why it is called "wai". Kung Fu is a discipline and considered to be "waigong 外功". You can also regard Taekwondo or Karate as a type of "waigong" discipline.

Disciplines that cultivate inner Qi are called "neigong 內功". With Qi Gong, you are primarily moving the energy inside the body with gentle movements, and you can close your eyes to do it. It is then an "internal" exercise. Qi Gong is "neigong 內功" energy.

What is "Wushu" (武術)? Is Wushu the same as Kung Fu? Wushu is a classic Chinese term for "Kung Fu". "Wu" means "military" and "shu" means art. Kung Fu is an art. Wushu consists primarily of boxing, weaponry and less Qi Gong. It cultivates external and internal Qi.

In traditional ancient Chinese cultures, famous masters resided in the mountains and they have many followers, disciples and family members. They name their forms after a special group or family name. It's most common to use their last name. Each "family" will have disciplines or forms that they are famous for. They might be more famous for certain forms, such as Kung Fu, boxing, weaponry or Qi Gong.

The spelling of the names may be similar or totally different, as they are translated according to the sound of the characters in simplified Chinese or traditional characters. In my teachings, Master Wu and I decided to use less Chinese terms that create confusion. However, it is helpful to understand what the other books say.

Forms of Qi Gong

There are hundreds of styles of Qi Gong that are based on two primary forms, each one created for their own purpose and benefits: Hard and Soft Qi Gong.

Hard Qi Gong includes anti-hitting, sleeping on needles or broken glass, breaking bricks and the spear to the throat, for example. This type of Qi Gong is what you see in movies or in public demonstrations. My teacher Master Wu also learned this form of Qi Gong, but believed it was dangerous to teach and would ultimately cause long term health problems.

Soft Qi Gong focuses on cultivating health, vitality and longevity by collecting "Universal Qi 宇宙氣" and strengthening our inner Qi. Soft Qi Gong consists of: Moving Qi Gong or Quiet Qi Gong.

Moving Qi Gong practice is a series of movements that are gentle, soft and promote balance and overall wellbeing.

Quiet Qi Gong promotes involuntary movements. The practice is done in a still and fixed position, usually standing with the arms positioned in a certain way. As the Qi moves effectively to the area that has blockages, the area will begin to move involuntarily, for example, hands, legs and even neck. The practitioner loses control of the Qi.

In China, according to Master Wu, Quiet Qi Gong is not promoted due to being regarded as unsafe to practice. I have never practiced it and cannot comment myself, but here is a real story of a student.

Mrs. Mak used to practice Quiet Qi Gong for a while and it helped her health improve. However, she didn't want to practice it anymore, because every day at a certain time, she felt her body wanting to move and she needed to go home and practice. If she didn't, she felt terrible and embarrassed as her body moved involuntarily. She needed at least 45 minutes to allow her body to finish its movements. Mrs. Mak began practicing Soft Qi Gong with us for about six months to clear the responses caused by Quiet Gong, and finally took charge of her own Qi.

As you can determine from the story, Quiet Qi Gong may cause some embarrassment, especially when you are around friends and family, and your body begins to move on its own when you would rather be quiet and calm. Quiet Qi Gong may not be good for those who are suffering from mental challenges too.

I encourage beginner students to focus on the breathing and movements to easily release their negative thoughts. If you wish to practice Quiet Qi Gong, I highly recommend that you seek lessons from very experienced instructors.

Soft, Moving and Medical Qi Gong are the three practices I focus on teaching. Our teachings focus on helping students to create the powerful Qi.

Medical Qi Gong

There are Qi Gong forms for improving health, which have not been researched; however, as more forms are researched and proven successful in helping general health - some support the healing process of certain illnesses in the body. Under these circumstances, Qi Gong is sometimes referred to as Medical Qi Gong, especially in China. There are also specialized Qi Gong forms designed for providing help with certain weaknesses or emotional issues in the body. In such cases, this is known as Prescribed Medical Qi Gong.

For example:

Qi Gong is like a happy pill

Qi Gong is like a painkiller

Qi Gong is like a sleeping pill

Qi Gong is an anti-aging pill

Medical Qi Gong and Diabetes

Joh Friedrich

I have been teaching Tai Chi and Qi Gong since 2000, including Medical Qi Gong. I'm continuing my learning process, because you never stop being a student. What I found with this particular form of Qi Gong is that it is a powerful one. I've been an insulin dependent diabetic for more than 40 years. This form of Qi Gong has helped me and I'm in better health than 20 years ago. So for anyone to learn this form, and wants to teach it, I think Master Teresa's program is excellent. I think it's a program that will give you new insights into the whole thinking of Tai Chi and Qi Gong, and the Chinese way of thinking about better health that our western world needs to learn more about. I hope I'm contributing to that.

When students practice Qi Gong for "big" medical reasons, such as cancer, they are encouraged to rest more and do less. There is a tendency to want to do more once they have more energy, for example, clean the house and engage in physical activities. If your objective is to heal the body, you need to rest the body and practice Qi Gong as much as you can. Conserve your energy so that the body has lots of power, or as they say in China "bullets" to conquer the health issue.

Qi Gong Is Not A Religion

If Qi means energy, it can also be thought of as *love energy*. When we practice Qi Gong, it is a way of loving ourselves; and a way of collecting the energy of creation. We can think of the Qi or love coming from the universe, nature and the earth. Students can ask their God to send Qi or send blessings, or love.

Some Qi Gong masters promote the esoteric, such as out-of-body experiences, which is not part of the normal teachings.

There are people who resist Qi Gong because they are afraid it conflicts with their religious beliefs. Qi Gong is not a religious practice. It is a practice of mindful breathing exercises usually with gentle movements for improving health. Why would people think so? One of the reasons is because of a scholar named Laozi, who was also a Qi Gong master. He was born around the 4th or 5th century BCE - equivalent to the period in Chinese we call "spring" or "autumn", or the warring period ("春秋戰國時代/春秋战国时代").

 It was a time of numerous schools of philosophies. Many famous scholars were born during this time and Laozi was one of them. His philosophical premise was Taoism or Daoism 道家, which was considered a religion in the China and Hong Kong regions. Laozi promoted the practice of Qi Gong for longevity and spiritual development.

My Qi Gong is taught without religion.

2. QI GONG ENDORSEMENTS

Giving individuals the power to determine and manage their own health and destinies is the secret of true healing.

- **Dr. Effie Poy Yew Chow**

Sharon Cass-Toole, PhD, DCEP

Integrative Psychotherapist and Wellness Consultant
Founder, Meridian Psychotherapy Services
Executive Director, Canadian Association for Integrative and Energy Therapies (CAIET)
Conference Director, Annual Canadian Energy Psychology Conference

Qi Gong is a foundational healing discipline and a powerful self-healing art. Learning and practicing Qi Gong will help you to gain mastery of yourself while awakening your healing abilities. It is the ancient art of effortless power that cultivates energy from the inside out. This practice is a fabulous resource to integrate the body, mind/emotion and spiritual energies.

Qi Gong (pronounced "chee-gung") is a 5,000-year-old traditional form of Chinese energy exercise for the body, mind, and spirit. It is a system for improving and maintaining health, as well as helping to cure disease. The basic aim is to bring the body into a state of balance and self-regulation. Qi Gong literally means "Breath Work" and is a distillation of several ancient healing systems. The practice of Qi Gong is based upon the cultivation and balance of Qi (or chi), generally translated as "Life Energy". This concept is at the core of every aspect of Chinese culture, including art, architecture, philosophy, sports and science.

Typically, a Qi Gong practice involves rhythmic breathing coordinated with slow stylized repetition of fluid movement, a calm mindful state and visualization of guiding Qi through the body.

Once a hidden practice, jealously guarded by the elite spheres of Classical Chinese society, and later forbidden by the Cultural Revolution, Qi Gong today enjoys vast popularity among the Chinese people, official support by the Chinese Ministry of Health, and intensive scrutiny by the Chinese scientific community. Qi Gong is one of Traditional Chinese Medicine's (TCM) principal methods of treatment. Though there are many schools and adaptations, the concurrent theories are the same in all of them.

Qi Gong is a discipline that anyone can learn. Many people practice Qi Gong simply because it makes them feel good, perform better, experience higher levels of energy and stamina, and reach their level of optimal health. Qi Gong can improve sports performance, prevent jet lag, and supercharge the immune system. Qi Gong practice has been shown to super-oxygenate the cells of the body. It can reduce stress, improve bowel function, and relieve the symptoms of insomnia and other sleep disorders. In the area of pain control, Qi Gong practice can relieve acute and chronic pain, reduce the pain of childbirth, and speed recovery from sports or other injuries. In addition, Qi Gong can increase the effectiveness of Western medications, may reduce the side effects and even allow the use of smaller doses. Many scientific studies have documented that Qi Gong has value in the treatment of more serious problems. It can reduce healing time after surgery by 50%, normalize the blood pressure, and heal tuberculosis. It can heal gastric and duodenal ulcers, chronic atrophic gastritis (stomach inflammation), and liver disease. It also has been effective nearsightedness (myopia) and improves mental performance. It also has been effective in the treatment of substance abuse, obesity, respiratory conditions, asthma, and allergies.

Benefits have also been seen in a long list of serious neuromuscular conditions, such as post-stroke syndrome, paralysis from brain and spinal cord injuries, multiple sclerosis, aphasia (loss of the power of expression of speech), Parkinson's disease, and Cerebral Palsy.

Qi Gong has been shown to reduce deaths related to high blood pressure, reduce the frequency for strokes, reduce the incidence of retinopathy (deterioration of the back of the eye), improve the efficiency of the pumping action of the heart, and decrease blood viscosity ("thin" the blood). It has also improved EKG (heart) and EEG (brain) readings, normalized hormonal levels and improved blood sugar levels in diabetics. In more than thirty research studies, Qi Gong has been found to reverse the effect of aging. Qi Gong will wake up your Chi, open your meridians and mobilize your healing energy, leaving you feeling alive and rejuvenated!
Qi Gong can help you:

- *Reduce stress and relax*
- *Be more joyful*
- *Increase energy*
- *Clear anxiety*
- *Alleviate insomnia*
- *Transform depression into inspiration*
- *Regulate body weight*
- *Reduce craving*
- *And much more*

Erin Dixon

Qi Gong Instructor, Qi Gong Fa Qi Si, Reiki Master, Yoga Instructor, Native Awareness Trainer (Toronto, Canada)

Gansie wo de weida de laoshi I gexinge!
A heart song of gratitude for my great teacher!

Close your eyes and take a slow, leisurely walk in a thriving old growth temperate rainforest in the Haida Gwaii. Vitality, wisdom and the presence of timelessness wash over you like great rains, and as you lie down in complete surrender on this forest floor, you return as the essence of mergence - the great ocean of Qi. Great mystery transforms into great clarity. This story line paints an expression of my experience being in Master Teresa's Qi Gong workshops.

On this great journey we are blessed with many teachers that rise and fall away, as the cycles of nature reflect on water. Then, there are the teachers whom you meet a great peace beholds you, in that a great tree of life has taken seed in your being and you are blessed to sit together. Master Teresa® has been this teacher for me. I had the opportunity to first meet Master Teresa® at her first class, following Grandmaster Wu's transition in early 2006, which gave me a unique experience of baring witness to the passing of the mission and lineage without comparison or expectation. The presence of the lineage before me felt - and still feels like - sitting in a room of pure gold. When I learned that Master Teresa® was returning to China to complete some of the work Grandmaster Wu started in Guangzhou province, I decided to follow the Qi and asked if I could join her. I was already traveling eastward during the same season. My respect and devotion to Master Teresa® as a teacher and her mission naturally flourished in the presence of her work in schools, in parks, communities, and with Grandmaster Wu's family and grand children.

Having the opportunity to be in the spaces and following the footsteps of Grandmaster Wu's journey, was enlightening. I listened to stories of how he came into awareness running through the forest around his family home and feeling the Qi fuelling his being. One of the greatest experiences was during a visit to his previous home, Master Teresa®, after teaching a Qi Gong practice, we went into his room and it felt as though our entire beings opened up like the sky. We were all in tears and in awe of his presence and Qi.

I have had the great opportunity to attend many different workshops, one-on-one healing sessions, teacher training courses with Master Teresa®, including the most recent Fa Qi training. I have been able to cultivate Qi Gong in every aspect of my life. From a personal daily practice to teaching classes in different communities and all ages, Qi Gong brings gifts on every level of being. Daily practice repaired my nervous system when doctors told me I would never be the same. My father said my health and energy is beyond anything he had seen even before I was out of balance.

Qi Gong taught me how to play the flute as a Spirit Player. In other words, surrender to the Qi to play the flute! Natural, untapped gifts rise to the surface. Qi Gong deepened my meditation and yoga practice, and as a growing Reiki master and teacher, practicing many different healing arts, the gifts of Master Teresa® and this lineage were crystal clear. People often ask what the difference is and I feel that experience is the greatest teacher. Ask your experience. We all love to see results: a butterfly's wings restored, a dog's eye healed, a gnarled, arthritic hand opens, an infection clears, tragedy lifts and a disease released with ease. Currently, I have the opportunity to work as a Native Awareness Trainer, in which I have the opportunity to facilitate different community initiatives, including youth programs. We incorporated Qi Gong into our traditional circles to help introduce some key aspects of Qi Gong, such as abdominal breathing and going inward to relax and open the body. We have also used Qi Gong at teacher training retreats and at First Nation community service providers' sharing circles. I can share that no matter the service or art you are providing to your community or family, Qi Gong will bring many unexpected gifts with one of the biggest being a deepened awareness of, presence and skills in all directions. I have found that the more I went inward to "clean up" as Master Teresa® would say, the deeper my Qi Gong practice became and the more I shared outwards, the true reflections of internal exercises.

One of the greatest treasures I feel is witnessing the sheer joy of service Master Teresa® holds in her mission to spread the empowering arts of Qi Gong. Even though Master Teresa's great teacher Grandmaster Wu transitioned, she continues to evolve in her own being and skill. This is a true teacher and Master.

"A Qi Gong Introduction"

During a women's fundraiser for Couchiching Jubilee House, a home for young single mothers in Orillia, I offered several introductory Qi Gong sessions for their annual Diva Day. As it was the first time all participants experienced Qi Gong, we focused on foundational aspects of posture, breath, awareness and relaxing the body. It was incredibly powerful to watch many ladies who sat down with chronic pain, headaches or exhaustion walk away with no pain after 20 minutes of Qi Gong! Being a completely new experience, they were very intrigued and empowered. It was very moving to observe them come to the realization that they have the ability to bring their own bodies into balance.

"Restoring From Anxiety"

I had the opportunity to share with a woman who suffered from anxiety and decided to treat her naturally. Being a young mother and a working professional, she gave herself little time for self-care. After an individual session, her strong determination and dedication led her to a daily practice in the morning before she started her day. This daily practice led to great results that she continues to share with me. Some of them include: being excited to wake up in the morning, a feeling of peace and relaxation as things arise, an increased sense of awareness and the nature of mind, and most of all, the feeling of empowerment. She continues to practice and live the results!

"Fa Chi Si Healing"

I have had the opportunity to begin my Fa Chi Si training with Master Teresa® and I am witnessing results on the physical level that I haven't seen working with other energy healing modalities. In the northern communities there are many dogs living freely and there are often fights between them. I had the opportunity to meet one who had just been in a fight and his eye was cut, red, swollen and bleeding. Immediately I had the sense from the dog to provide Fa Chi to encourage the healing process. My colleagues were with me so they witnessed the transformation. After the initial session, I kept meeting the dog and gave him sessions during the afternoon and into the evening. I wanted to see him as much as possible, because we were flying out the next day. Well in the morning my colleague called me outside and the dog's eye was quickly healing! The swelling and redness were gone and the gaping cut now was a small scab. I was blown away! Moreover, the spirit of the dog seemed to be in harmony! I use Fa Chi all the time with animals and with all forms of life, and I am always amazed at the results!

"Spiritual Soul Mate"

Everyone loves a love story. To top it off this is also a Qi Gong love story. Looking back I can see how the practice of Qi Gong naturally encouraged the connection to my partner, Adrian. We had originally met at a Yoga school in early 2005, and stayed friends for a few years, because he was living in the UK. We always need a little help from a friend and a teacher. When I was with Master Teresa® in China in the fall of 2006, I kept telling her about Adrian. She said to follow the energy and go to England to visit him and to be open to that energy - a deepening lesson. A few months later, Adrian joined me in northern Thailand and the next spring in India, and Nepal. I kept listening to the Qi and my heart. Having practicing Qi Gong, and being with Master Teresa®, it helped me to understand more about accessing the 'golden layer' of mind/being and let the Qi guide you. While on the plane to meet Adrian's family for the first time, all I could hear was "welcome home" resounding in the air. I already felt at home and heart with his family while in the airplane and upon the meeting. When Adrian came to Canada with me, it was the same.

In 2010, Master Teresa® blessed our wedding ceremony with her presence - the energy winds were magnificent and given the storms we felt incredibly calm and clear! Words cannot describe how lucky I felt for that level of support. One of the greatest gifts of our union is that we continue to evolve and grow into life together. We have also worked with Master Teresa in the couple's sessions, aimed to release, revitalize and restore, and through this experience gave us the opportunity to build more awareness - mindfulness and skill to care for the life cycles and harmony in our relationship. It is a natural way of life and being in the world and I really love participating in Adrian's Tai Chi classes and practicing Qi Gong, meditation and yoga together and supporting each other in energy balancing with Fa Chi Si or Reiki.

I continue to meet people from many different directions and no matter what arise from their experience, the practice and impact of regular Qi Gong practice on their life's synergistic alignment and pathway is crystal clear. Now 13 years of Qi Gong, I have witnessed many transformations from changes in career and aligning with purpose to releasing trauma, contraction and conflicting patterns. Regular practice naturally cleans and clears, builds and harmonizes our life force, and in so attracts and regenerates the true reflection and resonance of our being - a return to our true nature and the essence of the good life.

Dr. Elvis Ali
B.Sc, ND, F.I.A.C.A., RAc

THE BENEFITS OF QI GONG

For most of us, when we think about exercise, we associate it with losing weight or meeting some kind of physical fitness goal, but did you know that exercise is just as important for your mental health as it is for your physical body?

In fact, keeping your mind in great shape is one of the most important ways to keep your body in good health!

Qi Gong is one exercise that has helped me and my patients both physically and mentally to alleviate stress. It is not stress that affects us, causing detrimental results on our overall health, but rather, our reaction as well as our perception to stress. Our body tries to cope with stress, via nervous, endocrine, and immune systems. Qi Gong has been shown in studies as an adjunctive exercise therapy for older people with chronic conditions. Further, it is very effective at reducing fatigue, improving alertness and concentration, and at enhancing overall cognitive function. This can be especially helpful when stress has depleted your energy or ability to concentrate.

Exercise and other physical activity produce endorphins which are released in the brain, acting as a natural painkiller and helps improve the ability to sleep, which in turn reduces stress. The increase of endorphins in your body combats stress and produces feelings of euphoria, relaxes tense muscles and enhances immune response.

Qi Gong has been very effective in reducing stress perception, anxiety, anger, and improving the quality of life among many individuals. Scientists have found that regular participation In aerobic exercise has shown to decrease overall levels of tension, elevate and stabilize mood, improve sleep, and improve self-esteem. About five minutes of aerobic exercise can begin to stimulate anti-anxiety effects.

In our society, there is a lot of focus on body image. We all know if you exercise on a consistent basis, you'll likely shed a few pounds which can give you a great sense of accomplishment and affect how you feel about your body image. Qi Gong can be implemented daily as a regular exercise to decrease the tension levels, stabilize mood, improve sleep and improve self-esteem! It also results in higher energy levels which make you feel more positive, motivated and confident! All these positive results can help keep your mind in the right place and keep your body functioning the way it's naturally meant to.

I personally recommend 2 1/2 hours of moderate- intensity physical activity and 1 1/4 of vigorous-intensity activity per week.   In addition, one can take the time to practice Qi Gong on a daily basis for a few minutes and make the experience more enjoyable do something you love! There are lots of ways to get moving in our daily lives. For some it's the gym and for others it may be a quick jog outdoors, or even playing sports with some friends.

Qi Gong is very invigorating and as with any type of exercising, as long as you get your body moving it will help improve your body and mind, as well as give yourself some time for a little bit of fun!

Hon. Dr. Sheila McKenzie, RDH, PhD, IMD, DHS

Registered Dental Hygienist
Doctorate in Integrative Medicine
Homeopathic Medical Practitioner and Medical Acupuncturist
Integrative Medicine Practitioner, Doctor of Humanitarian Service
President WONM and Clinics for Humanity, IPSP
Deputy Minister of the National Assembly Canadian Parliamentary Group
Dame of Merit the Sovereign Order of the Orthodox Knights Hospitallers of St John of Jerusalem
Grand Prior of Humanitarian Medical Order of Knight Hospitallers (HMOKH) for North America
The World Organization of Natural Medicine (WONM) is an international non-profit, politically and religiously neutral humanitarian NGO
(Toronto, Canada)
https://www.integrativehealth.info/
https://www.wonm.org/

I'm an integrative medicine practitioner, specializing in oral and homeopathic medicines, and President of the World Organization of Natural Medicine. I can see that homeopathic medicine fits well with Qi Gong as they are both based on the energy systems of medicine. I also recommend this type of exercise of energy therapy to my own homeopathic patients as it is the best type of treatment.

I think that Master Teresa Yeung is doing a wonderful job and I recommend her work and this book for the betterment of humanity as a whole.

David Watson

Deep Trance Psychic, Ask the Willows, Life Strategist
(Toronto, Canada)
http://www.askthewillows.com

I first met Master Teresa Yeung about 10 years ago. It was at the time I was doing channel readings. I had a number of people coming to me for physical healing so I started sending them to Master Teresa® and her mentor, Master Wu. My channel source, The Willows, indicated that Master Teresa® and Master Wu would be the people to go to for physical healing. This happened ever so often over a few months. Then out of the blue, I received a call from Master Teresa®, thanking me for all the clients I was sending and how glad she was that they were able to help them. She wanted to give me a free process to meet her and Master Wu. Over time we became friends and sent people back and forth to each other so that they would benefit from both our gifts of healing. I also spent time learning the Qi Gong method from Master Teresa® and Master Wu and it really helped me a lot in balancing the energy in my body and with the hands-on healing which is part of what I do on a regular basis with my clients. The techniques are absolutely sensational.

I want to further relate a story that many people are not aware of. When Master Wu left the physical and crossed into spirit, I was called to his home and sat down with Master Teresa® and Madame Wu, to do a reading about what Master Teresa® should do next... That was the question: What to do next? We connected with Master Wu and Master Teresa® was given a lot of interesting information during that session. Master Wu again re-enforced that he wanted her to carry on the work they had begun and it was very important for her to teach the international style of Qi Gong in the west. Master Teresa® was not really thinking about continuing in that way. In fact, given the choice (through the reading) to take on the challenge - against all odds that a woman could be a master of a discipline that is historically bestowed upon a man, is remarkable. Particularly in the way that she has over the years, the organization continues to shift, change and grow, and has turned into something very beautiful and powerful.

Master Teresa® has stepped outside of tradition and stereotypes, and stepped into doing the work, and continues to bring Qi Gong to more and more people. It was important to pass on this information so that people have an appreciation that my friend Master Teresa® does what she does as a calling in life and that's the kind of energy that makes things happen. Thanks Master Teresa®, great knowing you and I look forward to years and years of our friendship growing even more.

3. NOTES FROM THE AUTHOR

Understanding The "Qi (Chi)" In Qi Gong

My teacher, Master Wu used to say, "Blood is the mother of the Qi." If you have blood, you have Qi. We all understand that if we have no blood, we will die. However, if we have no Qi, will we die? Yes, in Chinese we say that, "If you have no Qi, you are dead." We will look at a member of our family and say, "Your blood Qi is kind of low today".

When you think of what Qi is, you just have to change the word to "energy" and you will understand the teachings and testimonials in this book. For example, to interpret the sentence, "My Qi is low" becomes "My energy is low or I am feeling tired".

In English, we do not think about what energy is or where it comes from, because it is part of our makeup. It's like breathing – the natural inhalation and exhalation of the breath. So, if we start replacing the words "Qi (Chi)" with energy, we would not have to question whether it is there at all. It starts to make sense.

Qi is the basis of Chinese culture. It's the basis of Kung Fu, acupuncture, reflexology, herbal medicine, Feng Shui, food and everything. From the time we are children, we describe things as "good Qi" or "bad Qi". We will say, "This house has great Qi", meaning this house brings prosperity and health. Qi is our vital energy – the energy of life itself. It is the energy of creation. Qi is in all living organisms, plants and animals. Universal Qi is the original energy. All human beings are born with blood and Qi. Therefore, to practice Qi Gong is to work with life force energy.

If you were to visit a traditional Chinese medicine doctor, you will be diagnosed with a "pulse reading". The doctor puts his or her fingers on your wrist to listen to your signals coming from the meridians and diagnose the functions of the organs. The doctor will diagnose the quality and speed of the pulse to reflect your health condition.

Reading the tongue is another way of diagnosing the conditions of the body. Qi that does not flow well is often described as Qi stagnation. For example, when the kidney is weak, the kidney has stagnation. Qi stagnation or blocked Qi, negative Qi, bad Qi means the Qi is not good for health.

Furthermore, the Chinese doctor may describe the conditions of your health with terms like: damp, heat, wind, dryness, cool or even cold. All of these descriptions are interesting but confusing to most people unless you have spent some time studying Chinese medicines.

I have some knowledge of Chinese medicines, because I was using them for over 10 years before I started my Qi Gong journey. My pulse was so weak that doctors would sigh and shake their heads. They barely heard a pulse. Since practicing Qi Gong for some time now, they no longer disapprove of my pulse, because I am practicing Qi Gong to heal the root cause of my health issues. Practicing Qi Gong improves the flow of Qi energy, clears stagnation and balances the dampness, heat, wind and dryness of the body.

Qi means "energy" Gong means "work" or "practice". Qi Gong is a kind of internal exercise, which involves visualization, breathing, simple movements or no movement, using the mind to move the flow of Qi in the body. When the Qi flows, we have better health as we clear bad or stagnant Qi from the body. A simple analogy would be: a river is flowing downstream smoothly and one day, a mudslide happens and many rocks fall from the hillside into the river. The river still flows, but flows much slower. Later, there is another mudslide and the river flows even more slowly. When there is heavy rain, the level of water rises, the river flows better again. Another way to improve the flow of the river is to remove the rocks and soil. Or maybe in time, the water gradually washes some of the mud away.

If you look at the river as our bodies, the mud and soil are the blockages we face that impede optimal health. When our bodies are heavy, the flow of energy is good or blood circulation is good. If we fall down and get bruises, the bruises would be the mud. If we are hurt extensively, we will have more pain and even swelling. A new source of Qi that we can find from practicing Qi Gong is like adding water from upstream to help the water flow better downstream. The mud and rocks are still there, but the river flows better. When we do not practice, we will not feel well. We will only feel well when the mud and rocks are totally removed. This takes time, but it is possible. Time and dedication is needed. Finding a Qi healer is good, because the extra help from their Qi removes the blockages faster.

While there are thousands of forms of Qi Gong involving regular practice, discipline, and in most cases gentle physical movement, Qi Gong is not a sport, nor is it about competition. Rather, it is about supporting our health through focused relaxation, controlled breathing, and meditation.

Ultimately, Qi Gong is for all those who wish to take charge of, and to participate in, their own well-being. Because practicing Qi Gong makes you feel good, you will actually look forward to your practice.

The use of Qi Gong to improve health or even as a last resort to reverse incurable diseases is a belief system in the culture. The Chinese believe if you really practice Qi Gong or find a Qi Gong master to send you Qi, you have a better chance to survive certain diseases. In today's world, as we have better medicines, the use of Qi Gong for this purpose is declining. The search for better herbs and drugs, surgeries, invasive therapies are more accepted as the means to deal with diseases.

Practicing Qi Gong does not involve taking medicines, but the result from doing Qi Gong regularly often gives the results like taking medicine. For example, sleep better without the need to take sleeping pills; less pain and without the need for painkillers; breathe better without an asthmatic puffer. Qi Gong can be a painkiller, a sleeping pill and much more. Some people are looking for Qi Gong to help them fight a disease. Qi Gong does not fight. It harmonizes and balances. We are in charge of our own Qi. When Qi Gong gives health benefits, it is sometimes referred to as Medical Qi Gong, which is a term used in China.

Try this experiment before you start your Qi Gong journey: go to a mirror and look at your tongue. Look at it for colour and thickness. Make a note of what you see. When you start your practice, and assuming that you are doing everything right, such as eating healthy foods and practicing your Qi Gong properly, your tongue will start to look different as your circulation improves with the Qi practice. For myself, I can really see the difference in my tongue. Some students have used other methods to see the difference of their energy before and after a Qi Gong practice.

- *Live cell microscopy to look at the health of their live blood.*
- *Capture the readings of their bio-plasma fields or auras with a Kirlian camera.*
- *Digital infrared imaging before and after a Qi Gong practice. I have not done it yet, but I am sure it works wonderfully.*

Digital infrared imaging is being used as an alternative method to mammograms. Breast Thermography as it is known, checks the health of the breasts safely. There are huge concerns by holistic women that mammograms increase the risk for developing breast cancer and raise the risk of spreading or metastasizing an existing growth. This concern is based on the understanding that an X-ray poses cancer risks. Radiation emanating from mammograms can be 1,000 times greater than a chest X-ray. Digital infrared and self-examination are important; also the continuous balancing of Qi energy and sending Qi to the breast are important.

When one practices Qi Gong diligently and with the right teacher, we can develop extraordinary abilities too. The abilities include sending Qi out, feeling the Qi of the students, do remote healing and are able to scan and know what and where a student's physical and emotional challenges are. My teacher used to scan the people's body and was able to tell where the blockages were. I have also developed this ability and I am developing programs to pass these teachings on to my students.

Our body needs to know what we are trying to achieve or accomplish. Each movement has meaning. If a teacher explains why you are doing the movements, this will help you have better results. Learning a new form of Qi Gong is like driving to another place. Where do you want to go or achieve? In the world, most people want to look younger, healthier, stronger and happier. When we eat well, take herbs, buy creams, etc., usually we are trying to take things into the body to have an effect on our wellbeing, looks or health. We can say that this is the result of fixing the **outside in**. When we practice Qi Gong, we are doing the opposite: working from the **inside out**, which means we eat nutritious food, take supplements and exercise. By practicing Qi Gong, we improve the Qi and energy flow to the organs, glands, to obtain health, strength, youthfulness and longevity. Balancing the flow of Qi, we will become more emotionally balanced, thus become happier.

Good and Bad Qi

It's not so much that there is good or bad Qi in our body. Bad energy (negative energy) can be explained as stagnant energy in the body. A quick example would be gas, lactic acid, cysts and fibroids, etc. Or we can say when our eyes are tired, the eyes have weak Qi or are injured.

What's important is the need to be balanced and in harmony by moving the energy. Going for a leisure walk is a way of moving the energy. In Qi Gong, we use the mind and gentle movements to move the energy more efficiently for homeostasis. Often, we will visualize breathing in good energy and exhaling out negative energy as a means of letting go.

Oxygen, Cancerous Cells and Qi Gong

In 1931, Dr. Warburg won his first Nobel Prize for proving that cancer is caused by a lack of oxygen respiration in the cells. He stated in an article entitled, *The Prime Cause and Prevention of Cancer* that the "cause of cancer is no longer a mystery. We know it occurs whenever any cell is denied 60% of its oxygen requirements".

In August 2009, scientists from the Cancer Research Department at MRC Gray Institute for Radiation Oncology and Biology at the University of Oxford, published that cancer cells low in oxygen are three times more resistant to radiotherapy. By restoring oxygen levels to that of a normal cell, the tumors become three times more sensitive to treatment. Even better, more stable blood supply in the tumor enables improved delivery of chemotherapy drugs. Clinicians were excited by this discovery and planned to expand trials to more research, bringing new hope to patients.

In Qi Gong, we primarily focus our practice on how to breathe in air slowly, evenly and deeply. Thus opening the lung allows the body to take in more oxygen and oxygenate the cells. Qi Gong is indeed a great tool for cancer patients.

Athletic Performance and Qi Gong

Qi Gong is the base of Kung Fu. A Kung Fu master practices how to improve their body's flow of energy to be stronger in their physical strength and power in combating. There has been research in China that states, practicing Qi Gongs raises the level of testosterone and balance hormones. Qi Gong definitely speeds up the recovery of injuries. Other benefits include calming the mind, loosening up tightness, and building better breathing and clearing the build-up of lactic acid from a workout. I find, because athletes are young and have vibrant energy, under guidance, they respond quickly to Qi Gong.

Oxygen, Light and Qi Gong

When we breathe, we breathe in oxygen; however, it's not just oxygen. We also bring in the light and light has colours. Light wraps itself around the oxygen molecule. Oxygen and light are good energy, which we live on and cannot do without. When we practice Qi Gong, we breathe and bring in air and light to oxygenate our cells.

Practitioners can visualize bringing in universal Chi during practice and just thinking of bringing in the light too.

功夫太極為基礎

Kung Fu and Tai Chi build a good Qi Gong foundation.

The Difference Between Tai Chi and Qi Gong

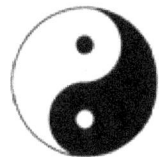

Tai Chi - also known as Tai Chi Chuan or Taiji Quan 太極 or 太极) - means, "Infinite Changes". It is a Chinese term that represents the Yin/Yang symbol and is considered slow motion Kung Fu. This symbol represents two fishes (one for Ying and one for Yang) and it is also the symbol of Taoism. Like all forms of Kung Fu, it consists of cultivating the inner life force Qi energy. Practicing Tai Chi has many health benefits. Qi Gong and Tai Chi are both Chinese traditions that increase our life force energy through exercises. These exercises promote circulation and personal energy for self-healing and wellbeing. You might have seen people practicing them in parks and community centers.

The Chinese practice Tai Chi for general health maintenance is like practicing Yoga: while if someone is suffering from a major disease like cancer, one can immediately turn to Qi Gong instead of Tai Chi. Chinese believe that practicing Qi Gong and receiving Qi from a Qi Gong master may save their lives.

Tai Chi movements involve the gentle movements of extending and lifting the arms, legs and hands. Qi Gong is simpler. It has fewer movements and easier to practice in slow motion. There are different forms of Tai Chi and Qi Gong exercises. All these different exercises have one thing in common: they vary the load on joint surfaces, increasing the flow of natural lubricants and nutrients to the joints, so they move more easily and freely. The exercises train the lung to inhale more oxygen and exhale carbon dioxide effectively. The exercises have proven to help boost the immune system, supporting our self-healing ability. Clinical research has been done on the practices of Qi Gong and Tai Chi on their healing benefits around the world.

Many people are also using these practices for reducing stress, as well as for specific health issues such as: shortness of breath, fatigue, fibromyalgia, pain, digestive problems, diabetes, blood pressure, headaches and auto-immune problems. It is particularly important to note that there is actually a Qi Gong exercise designed for vision. In 1990, Master Wu led a 100-healthcare professional team on Wu's Eye Qi Gong® research studies and went through 4,000 medical research studies in China. The same studies were repeated for three years on the same 4,000 people and had a proven success rate of over 90 percent!

The Wu's Eye Qi Gong® form is now used to support the healing of all kinds of eye problems: fatigue, pain, headaches, migraines and insomnia, and also is an immune booster.

If you are interested in knowing more about this topic, you will appreciate reading *The Harvard Medical School Guide to Tai Chi: 12 Weeks to a Healthy Body, Strong Heart, and Sharp Mind* written by Peter Wayne, PhD.

Tai Chi Instructor

I have been teaching Tai Chi for six or seven years and have been practicing it myself for more than 12 years. I was diagnosed with fibromyalgia and I was taking medication for sleep and pain to be able to control it. When I started Qi Gong about a year ago with Master Teresa® and infused myself with the breathing and the way to meditate that Master Teresa® is teaching, I stopped taking the medication! I'm able to sleep and the pain really went down quite a lot. I've been developing in Tai Chi my flexibility and balance, coordination and a new outlook to my life. However, Qi Gong has given me a different dimension – another dimension to teaching that I'm sharing with my students and I enjoy that very much. I would like to give this experience to as many students as possible, because it is really wonderful!

-     **Vera Stern, Qi Gong & Tai Chi Instructor**

Emotions and Qi Gong

In Chinese medicines, energy or Qi flows through the meridians (also known as channels). These meridians or channels create an energy map throughout the body. The energy is electromagnetic. Our organs are connected to the meridians. We believe that emotions are stored in the organs. You can look at different emotions as a certain kind of Qi, for example: happy Qi, fearful Qi, angry Qi or grief Qi. When we have resentments or anger, it is believed that the angry Qi energy is stored in the liver. When we overly care for others, we use our Heart Qi. When we worry, we deplete our Qi in the kidneys, weakening the physical kidneys. Through our practice of Qi Gong, we balance the emotions and replenish our organs and parts of our body.

As healthcare professionals and healers, we are more aware of the power of Qi, acupuncture points, meridians and how they support the healing of the body.

You may want to learn about my #1 International Bestselling book "Unlocking Your Happiness Within: Living the Life You Choose with Chi Gong". It has a book and workbook:

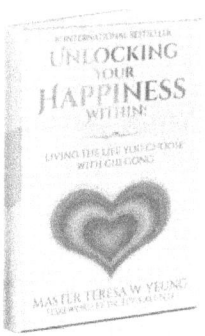

http://getbook.at/UnlockingYourHappinessWithin
http://getbook.at/Workbook_UYHW

How the Weather Affects Our Emotions

Because we are emotional and social creatures, we are affected by the weather. When it's sunny, we feel good, so our moods are better. When it's cloudy and rainy, we become tired and moody, not to mention if it's a stormy day.

The body makes Vitamin D when we are exposed to the sun. In the summer, when there is lots of sun, we tend to have fewer colds. That is why for many who believe in healing naturally, will triple their doses of Vitamin D in the winter to prevent getting the flu. (Please research this subject more yourself.) Certain research published that sunlight increases serotonin levels, which in turn makes us happier. For some people, if they find that during the winter season, they feel depressed or tired, it may be due to the lack of sunshine.

Practicing Qi Gong outdoors is preferred to enjoy the sunlight. However, practitioners can also practice Qi Gong indoors and visualize collecting sunshine in their practice. The practice of Qi Gong can help our adaptability to changes in the weather, build our immune system and keep us in a good mood. People with seasonal depression may also feel better using a light therapy lamp.

EMFs, Earth and Qi Gong

Radiofrequency Electromagnetic Fields (RF-EMF)

Wi-Fi signals use a frequency of 2.4 GHz, nearly identical to the frequency of microwave ovens (2.45 GHz) and similar to those of mobile or cell phones (GSM phones use 1.8 or 1.9 GHz and the UMTS 3G phones use 2.1 GHz). Sun frequencies are 2.5 times stronger than 50 years ago. Radiation coming from cell phones, Wi-Fi, laptops and microwave ovens can be called radiofrequency electromagnetic fields (RF-EMF). When I scan a body's energy field, EMFs feel like invisible lasers continuously cutting through our energetic bodies.

In recent years, there has been growing health concerns around the world as to whether EMF exposure is linked to many of today's unexplainable health problems; for example: nervous system disorders, sleep problems, chronic pain, anxiety, depression, headaches, brain cancer and fertility problems.

There are reports of decreasing sperm count and motility in men and, at least in the United States and Europe, new research says male infertility is getting worse according to studies in 2018. Factors attributed to this include exposure to pesticides, other hazardous substances, and RF-EMF.

https://www.ncbi.nlm.nih.gov/pmc/articles/PMC6240172/

Some people like me will remove electronic equipment from the bedroom for better sleep, or at least take them away from near the bedside. The best distance between you and electronics is at least 2.5 feet. I will definitely avoid using wireless computers and telephones and instead, I would use a landline. If it is possible, turning off the router cable box at night is also an effective strategy to reduce RF-EMF.

Wi-Fi energy is like microwave radiation, so why would I bring microwave energy to my ears which will go then into the brain? Earphones are still leading EMF radiation to the ears so turn on the speakerphone to talk. Another option is to use a protective shield which will decrease the RF-EMF and I have started to carry specific handmade EMF shields in my online store.

The practice of Qi Gong is more important than ever as it will help you to ground the energy of EMF and the disruptive solar energy. You train through Pureland Qi Gong® system to become a better antenna to attract positive energy and ground the negative energy.

A daily practice of Qi Gong - twice a day - is a good way to clear the EMFs and also "repair" any damage of EMFs on our bodies; I see it as healing the "holes".   For those who spend a lot of time on their cell phones, they can consider practicing the Ear Qi Gong. For those people that need to look at the computer monitor for many hours at a time, they can consider practicing the Eye Qi Gong for eye health, headaches, focus, better sleep and brain related issues.

There are many resources that provide good EMF protection products online. If you are choosing something a pendant, please make sure that the products allow you to reverse and still work. Some manufacturers do not tell you which side is the right side to face up. I saw one pendant which was quite expensive with the manufacturer logo on one side and the flower on the other side. I actually checked the energy and then found out that manufacturer logo has to be facing up and not the flower. You must check. I personally like this company: https://photonorgone.co.uk/

A Wonderful Reliever of Anxiety, Depression and Stress

There is a lot of stress in the world – from financial worries over the economy, fears over political instabilities, as well as concerns about the environment and the safety of our food and water. Even if we are not directly focused on these stressors, many people are impacted by the negative energies that come from other people's worries and concerns.

Stress is the result of how the body interprets messages. For many, these disruptive energetic vibrations related to stress can be very erratic and cause some degree of disorientation and uncertainty. People under stress may feel lost, not certain where they are in their lives, or where they should be headed. Unresolved feelings like these can cause emotional and physical health problems. In fact, studies have shown that various types of chronic stress are linked to a greater risk of heart disease and heart attacks.

Chronic stress can cause problems by elevating levels of adrenaline and adrenal steroid hormones. One homeopathic paper compared adrenalin arousal to "leaving a car engine idle at high speed." Even a simple argument can cause our hearts to beat faster, and our blood pressure to rise. Stress can also lead to depression and disturbed sleeping patterns, which can create other health issues. Stress is also not just an individual matter, it can have a negative effect on friends and family - anyone in personal contact with the stressed person can be adversely affected.

Smoking, Drinking Alcohol, Stress, Addiction and Qi Gong

I have seen students after practicing Qi Gong quit smoking, stop their cravings and even reduce alcohol consumption to much less too. It is all about how to manage your stress levels. The practice of Qi Gong is a great way to distract your feelings towards craving. Practice every time you have a craving for the wrongs.

There is a Pilot Study of Qi Gong for Reducing Cocaine Craving Early in Recovery published in Pub Med Central, 2013.
https://www.ncbi.nlm.nih.gov/pmc/articles/PMC3576894/

QI GONG AND OTHER HEALING MODALITIES

Acupuncture and Qi Gong

Qi is the basis for Chinese medicines. Inserting needles in different acupoints on the body's meridians or channels is called acupuncture. These channels can be described as invisible pathways in which the Qi flows throughout the body. In recent years, Qi Gong has increased in popularity after Tai Chi, because it has often been described as "acupuncture without needles." Acupuncture treatments based on Qi theory are being accepted as an effective way of treatments. A daily practice of Qi Gong improves the flow of our life force or energy throughout the body.

An acupuncturist can learn how to send Qi to any part of the body while using the needles. Patients may also take Chinese herbal medicines while having acupuncture treatments, which is the original way of Chinese healings. In addition, patients can also practice Qi Gong movements to enhance the flow of Qi at home and continue taking acupuncture treatments at the same time.

Dowsing, BioGeometry and Qi Gong

I remember in one of my classes, I saw one of my students, who is very experienced in dowsing, exclaim: "The Qi carries the gold frequency!" I saw the gold pendulum she was holding swing high, wide and strong around the area we were sending out Qi. Her excitement interested me!

A couple of years ago, when I was a speaker at an Energy Psychology Conference, I had the opportunity to learn about Dowsing and BioGeometry in the lectures. I came to understand how the ancient and wise Egyptians built homes, buildings and pyramids on special energy spots. The best sacred harmonic frequency is called, "gold frequency" and I was told that it's hard to find. People who carry gold frequency can be ascended masters.

In BioGeometry, it's being referred to as "BG3", which is highest form of energy quality producing harmony in the divine laws of nature. It's believed that the energy of these power spots have holistic healing properties, acting on the physical, vitality, emotional and mental levels. Sacred spots in the world carry these properties. It's believed that when someone sits in an environment with gold frequency, it will improve health and wealth for the best harmony.

I am very happy to let you know that Qi is the gold frequency and when you practice Qi Gong, you are creating the gold frequency. When you improve your Qi, you emit that Qi (gold frequency) to the environment and improve the energy in your environment. For those who know how to dowse for gold frequency, you can dowse the hand of Qi healers, dowse your Qi Gong T-shirts, DVDs and you will become excited by your findings.

Healthy Food and Qi Gong

Poor digestion does not allow the body to absorb the best nutrition of the food. Even if the food is healthy or organic, we still need to digest them. Qi Gong practice improves digestion, thus getting the most out of the value of our foods.

Meditation and Qi Gong

A great number of people, when exploring spiritual development, want to learn how to meditate. However, some find it very difficult, because thoughts keep arising in the mind. Qi Gong is like a moving meditation and can be a stepping stone to those who wish to meditate successfully. The reason is when we practice Qi Gong we focus on the movements and breathing techniques, performing a gradual habit to calm the mind.

Medicines and Qi Gong

Medicines often have side effects. On any drug prescribed, there is a long list of side effects. Qi Gong relaxes the body and promotes circulation. It is common for students to report that side effects are lessened with a Qi Gong practice. As the body strengthens, dosages of certain types of medications can be reduced or cancelled.

Science and Qi Gong

Qi Gong involves breathing and visualization techniques. Qi Gong's energy is bio-magnetic. When we breathe, our target is to work on slowing down the breath to four breaths a minute. Breathing in oxygen is healthier, as it provides what the body needs, or shall I say what the heart needs; another way to say it: "We are oxygenating our cells."

Research scientists love finding the answers to the unknown. I was introduced to one of James Oschman's book *Energy Medicine: The Scientific Basis by* one of my students in Florida. Dr. Oschman is a cellular biologist and physiologist who wrote a number of books on the mind-body connection and the role of "natural energies" for healing.

The work of Dr. Oschman is very important, because his books cover most of the questions people ask about the workings of energy, especially how it heals the body. With scientific evidence and research, for example, in medicine, magnetic from electricity, brain waves, bio-magnetic fields, cell structure, living matrix, acupuncture and related therapies, show that energy fields can be projected from the hands in Qi Gong, homeopathy, distant healings and group healing circles.

He explained in his book: *Molecules and their vibrations orchestrate all living processes. No one has ever seen a molecule: they are simply too small. Molecules are composed of atoms, which are made up of electrons. Virtually all of our knowledge about molecules, and about matter in general, has come from studying the ways light interacts with electrons. When two objects have similar natural frequencies, they can interact without touching."* On page 82 he states, *"Research shows that masters of the Qi Gong technique can project measurable amounts of heat from their palms to increase cell growth, DNA and protein synthesis, and cell respiration. One explanation for facilitation and inhibiting Qi is based on the fact that the circulation to the skin is influenced by the autonomic nervous system.*

View research articles: https://purelandqigong.com/articles/

Reiki and Qi Gong

Reiki 靈気 is a complimentary energy healing therapy founded by Mikao Usui (1965 -1926). Mikao Usui was born in Taniai, Japan and studied Shintoism, Buddhism, Taoism. In his memoir, it states that he travelled to China, the US and Europe in search of the power of natural healings. Later, Mikao fell into a trance and had an awakening, and found "Reiki" - a hands-on healing. Unfortunately, due to the 2nd World War, much of the original Reiki documents were lost.

As acupuncture and Chinese medicines are becoming popular and proven to be successful in healing, more Reiki masters are turning to Qi Gong to take them to the next level of awakening. Over 80 percent of students have heard of Qi Gong or took Reiki classes.

The practice of Qi Gong can enhance the work of Reiki. Qi Gong helps Reiki practitioners cleanse their Qi and replenish their life force energy. The techniques in balancing the Qi, using Qi Gong is very different to Reiki healing, because it is based on improving the flow of the Qi acupoints, meridians or channels with different visualization techniques. Qi Gong practitioners emphasize the need for a daily Qi Gong practice to enhance their ability to channel energy from the universe, protect the energy from loss and store or "bank" it in the body for future use. Students in our class commented on seeing the colour of channeled Qi Gong energy to be white or violet, which is different to Reiki energy.

Reiki Master

I've been practicing Reiki since 2002, and I've been a teacher since 2005. Grand Master Usui, the founder of Reiki as we know, was a practitioner of Kiku and master of Qi Gong. So you can see that someone who has created Reiki has a foundation within the Qi Gong practice. Qi Gong has many benefits in that you are cultivating energy. So it not only helps with the amount being given to heal others through your Reiki practice, or to facilitate the healing, it also helps to clear and ultimately gives more energy for strength. Also it gives you a level of awareness that is needed as a practitioner of what becomes giving away your energy. I have met many practitioners who felt depleted or felt that they picked up certain things, because they were not ready or didn't have the awareness of the boundaries and what was taking place. Qi Gong practice can give you lots of experience that will help in many different ways in your Reiki practice.

- **Erin Dixon, Qi Gong, Fa Chi Si, Reiki Master, Native Awareness Trainer**

Vibrational Therapies and Qi Gong

Vibrational medical techniques are acupuncture, homeopathy, gem and flower essences, colour, light and laser healing sound therapies, Reiki, Qi Gong and hands-on healing.

The word vibration or frequency refers to the pulsations of energy that makes up and patterns in all life and matter. Vibrations of atoms create sound and heat. Colour is being emitted when an object vibrates with the electrons of light. Each colour has its own vibrational frequency.

In Qi Gong, we use sounds and visualize colours for healing. Practitioners may actually feel a gentle vibration in their practice.

Final thoughts. . .

Qi is free. Qi is love. The practice of Qi Gong is the most inexpensive way of healing, and it is the light in darkness. You can imagine bringing the light of Qi into your body and visualize sending the heaviness, stress, illness, darkness inside you out of your body into the universe. Remember the energy of the universe is huge and your negative energy is so small. If you are struggling with health problems, practice Qi Gong two to three times a day and it will bring in more positive Qi energy into you. It is very simple to do and gives good results. Watch your thoughts as they are very powerful.

Lynne McTaggart's book, **The Intention Experiment** is an interesting exploration of the science of intention, and includes findings from leading scientists from around the world. The discovery demands that we pay better attention to our thoughts, intentions and actions.

There is a simple adage that says: "Thoughts become things." Put another way, we can say: "Wherever we put our focus that is our experience". A very simplistic example would be thinking of a friend and suddenly we receive a call or an email from him or her.

With empirical evidence that shows our mind as a powerful instrument to channel our thoughts, technologies are following suit to support this fact:

> At the 2010 Winter Olympics in Vancouver, British Columbia, there was a demonstration on thought-controlled lighting. People were asked to put on headsets and think of themselves increasing the brightness of lights on Toronto's CN Tower, Ottawa's Parliament Buildings and Niagara Falls.

Primitive mind-control is already used in games, such as Mattel's Mindflex, in which you wear a brainwave-reading headband and concentrate to raise and lower a ball held in mid-air by jets of air that respond to your brainwaves. If you research this subject, the news stated that IBM predicts that mind-controlled computers will be on the market within five years.

In 2013, biomedical engineers (three females and two males), at the University of Minnesota's College of Science and Engineering, determined for the first time that humans were able to successfully control the flight of flying robots using just their thoughts from a non-invasive skull cap. Bin He, lead author of the study and biomedical engineering professor, explained that this research is intended to help people who are paralyzed or have neurodegenerative diseases regain mobility and independence. The researchers said the brain - computer interface system works due to the geography of the motor cortex - the area of the cerebrum that governs movement. When we move, or think about a movement, neurons in the motor cortex produce tiny electric currents. Thinking about a different movement activates a new assortment of neurons. Sorting out these assortments laid the groundwork for the brain-computer interface.

I am indeed grateful to the scientists and researchers for their findings that support the "visualization techniques" used in our Qi Gong practice. They recognize the importance of the techniques and that they work. In our Pureland Qi Gong®, we focus on setting intentions to achieve the best results in all our Qi Gong exercises, including performing distant healings.

Here is a dialogue with a request for help.

Sunday evening

Client: *Hello Master Yeung. I am reaching out to you, because my daughter was in a horrific accident. She has suffered severe brain trauma, which was worsened even further by a stroke caused by the initial injury. We were wondering if you could use your masterful healing energy to help heal our loved one at her bedside in hospital. Thank you!*

Master T: *If you take a photo of her and send it to me please so I can read the energy. (I received a photo, and on Monday, I did a remote session.)*

Client: *Oh my goodness! Thank you so much! They are saying she is doing good and she actually breathed on her own for a couple of hours.*

(Tuesday, I received another message)

Client: *Dear Master Yeung, the CT scan shows the bleeding in her brain has gotten a bit worse. Tomorrow could you please focus your healing energy mostly on her brain and eyes? Thank you.*
(I asked some of my student practitioners to send Chi remotely to expedite healing.)

(Wednesday, I wrote her.)

Master T: *I did a remote session on her. Hope it helps. Pray.*

Client: *Thank you very much for your healing of my daughter. After a CT scan this morning, she is cleared for blood thinners from the stroke department and the neurological team!!! The vessels in her neck are also looking better! This is such positive news for us. Thank you for being a part of our journey.*

Master T: *Does this mean the bleeding in the brain stopped too?*

Client: *The neurological team said that it appears to have stopped!!*

(Following Monday, client reported that her daughter's condition remains stable.)

Qi, Chi or Ki Is The Key of Life

Believe it or not, the use of Qi Gong has no limit. To me, the sky is the limit. When you think, you are moving the Chi. I would even call the mind – the Chi. When you change the energy with Qi Gong practice, you release stuck energies, you also naturally or gradually change the prospective of life. You are more in love with yourself and compassionate about giving kindness and love to others. We sincerely wish *Life Force* will help your journey be easier and make a difference in your life.

We sincerely welcome you to join Pureland International Qi Gong™   and become one of our practitioners making a difference.

Great blessings to you 祝福你幸福快樂 **!**

Teresa Yeung

GENERATIONAL MASTER
OF CHI GONG

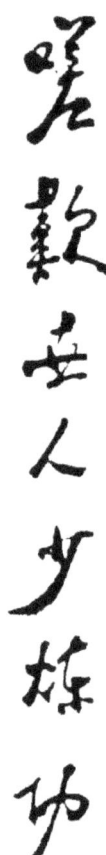

It is regretful that few people in the world are practicing Qi Gong.

4. MASTER WU WEI ZHAO (1933-2006)

My teacher was a very humble, kind and strong person. He did not like to boast about himself or let people know that what he did was special in his life. I knew that he would rather have me leave him alone than talk about his story. However, I felt the world deserved to honor his teachings to mankind. Here is the story that I can best remember from his documents:

Wu Wei Zhao 吳偉昭 was born in China. When Wu was a young boy he was inspired by his famed uncle, who practiced Kung Fung and Qi Gong. He once saw his grandmother picking up a kitchen knife and fought off a robber who came to the house. He was fascinated by the power of Kung Fu. At that time in the neighbourhood, there was a Master Sung, teaching Kung Fu. Every day after school, he would go to the place where they practiced and watched the adults happily practicing. Master Sung observed him and was touched by his love of the martial art and accepted him as a young student. He was only six or seven years old at the time.

Wu was a born leader, protecting the weak from being teased and harassed in his neighbourhood from the bullies when he was young. As a young boy, he helped in his father's fabric store. In China in those days, you closed the store by moving big heavy wooden doors one by one to lock up. Wu had great strength and could lift the doors with one arm, surprising all the adults. Wu was a natural athlete. As a young man, he was selected by the Chinese Government to learn different kinds of western sports from international coaches. He learned western fencing, swimming, gymnastics, track and field and bodybuilding from famous instructors from Russia, Hungary, Germany and Italy, invited to teach in China. During the intense personal training, muscle injuries became a problem. For that reason, his interest expanded to using Qi Gong energy to heal his own injuries, and clear up all the aches and pains in his body.

In China the best teachers are often found in temples in the mountains such as Tai Shan, Lo Shan, Wu Dang, to name a few. Each mountain represents a particular school. Wu traveled throughout China on a quest to find these teachers. Meeting up with various masters, he fine- tuned and trained himself while sharing his knowledge at the same time. As his reputation grew, many other secluded masters came directly to honor Wu and to pass on their knowledge to him, and in turn, he passed on his knowledge back to those who came to him.

He became a Master of over 100 Kung Fu techniques, soft and hard Qi Gong, Tai Chi and Wushu (a style of Kung Fu distinct to the northern region of China). In Wushu, he enjoyed practicing southern boxing, the praying mantis and anti-hitting, hard Qi Gong, and long range. In weaponry, he enjoyed practicing 10-foot long stick, double butterfly swords and three-section staff. He studied Qi Gong with many families, including Wu Dang, Shaolin, Omei and the Royal Family. In Tai Chi, he became a master of four famous Tai Chi families: Wu, Yang, Sun and Chan.

He was a Master of Western Fencing and co-founder of the first Western Fencing Association in Guangdong Province and in Guangzhou City. He was a referee, judge, arbitrator and the Director of the Opening Ceremony for the Chinese National Sports Competitions; a Kung Fu Master and Martial Arts Adviser of the Guangzhou City Chinese Martial Arts Association. He was the Vice-President of the Guangdong Province Zhineng Association. Zhineng Qi Gong is sometimes referred to as "Chi-lel" Qi Gong in North America. He was the Qi Gong Master in the Guangdong Province Physical Athletic Sports Hospital.

He introduced Qi Gong to national athletes. He taught hundreds of athletes medical Qi Gong and used external Qi to treat more than 300 kinds of illnesses and injuries. Some of his major accomplishments began in the mid 80's when he headed a medical team at the Qi Gong Centre of Guangzhou City Primary and Secondary Physical Education Health Research Association, and the Board of Education. He started clinical trials and research studies on the application of medical Qi Gong to heal illnesses and injuries for thousands of people. On the academic side, Master Wu was an educator, involved in educational work for 36 years in Guangzhou City. Then he graduated from Guangzhou City Teachers' College with top honors and was the honoree, invited to stay in the College and become a teacher, training future teachers. For 21 of those years, he was involved in developing educational policy, books, physical education and health work on the Board of Education in Guangzhou City. The students in the schools now are still practicing some of the exercise routines that he designed for physical education in China.

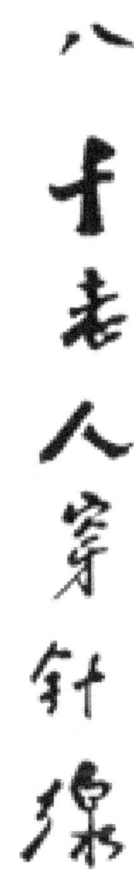

*An eighty-year-old woman was able to thread a needle through
practicing Qi Gong.*

In the late 1980s, Wu returned home from a trip and found his mother's eyes bleeding. It was diagnosed as a stroke and there was hardening of the arteries. According to the doctor, his mother was going blind. It would take years for the eyes to heal and the chances were slim. The Wu's Eye Qi Gong ® form was created overnight for healing his mother's failing eyes and kept her from going blind. Wu taught his mother his new Wu's Eye Qi Gong ® and also did intensive Qi healing on her eyes daily. In weeks, his mother's eyes regained complete vision and afterwards she could put a thread through a needle in her 80's. This was a real surprise to him and to the medical doctors.

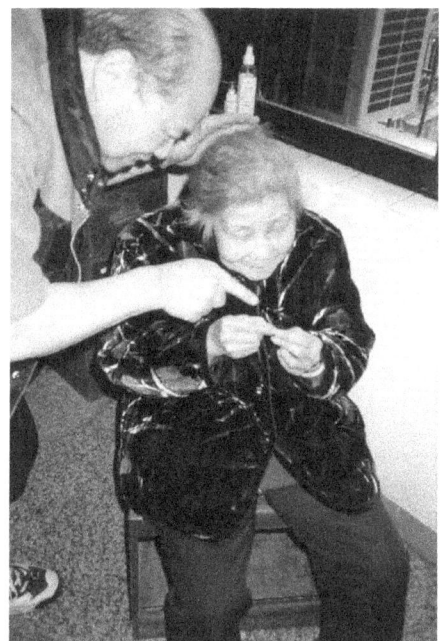

Later, the **Wu's Eye Qi Gong** ® was introduced to the public-school system in China. From 1990 to 1992, Wu represented the Guangdong Province and Guangzhou City and led a 100-person medical team to perform a three-year repetitive scientific research study on 4,000 people to use Wu's Eye Qi Gong ® to heal eye problems.

Wu's Eye Qi Gong® proved to have over a 90 percent success rate. Due to its success, Wu's Eye Qi Gong® was introduced throughout China to physicians and educators.

His Eye Qi Gong received many honors and awards:

- 1991- Guangdong Province Board of Education Award
- 1992- Guangzhou City Physical Education and Science Association Award
- 1992 - Guangzhou City Primary School Physical Education and Health Research Association Award

To this day throughout China, children in schools maintain a daily routine of eye exercises. Thanks to Master Wu, his research findings were officially published, including a Qi Gong thesis on *Use of Qi Gong to Prevent Myopia* and *Use of Qi Gong 311 Clinical Cases and Diseases*.

In 1993, his Qi Gong research studies were presented to the medical conference of physicians and doctors from Guangdong Provincial Preventive Medical Association. His Qi Gong was recognized and proven successful by various bodies of the government, including the physical, scientific research, medical and educational associations of the government of China. In 1995, Wu was invited to become a member of the Chinese Qi Gong Talent Bank "中國人才庫" of the Science Research Academy of Chinese Qi Gong "中國氣功科學研究會交流服務中心" (The Chinese Talent Bank is the highest official organization in the Qi Gong Network, organized and managed by the Exchange Service Center of the Science Research Academy of Chinese Qi Gong.)

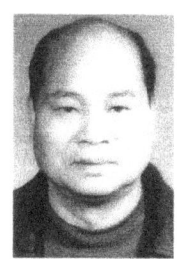

中国气功人才库由中国气功科学研究会组建，为我国最高级气功人才网络系统。它由中国气功科学研究会交流服务中心主办和管理。各级气功组织的会员和具有助理气功师以上职称的人员应为其必然成员，具有一定气功专长的人员也可自荐入库。入库人才将被国家优先选拔重用。人才库通信地址：北京 199 信箱中气交流服务中心。电话：8503551 或 8538785。

发现人才----选拔人才----重用人才

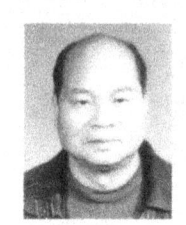

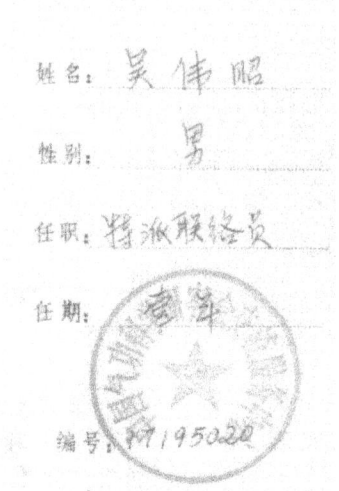

聘任单位：

中国气功科学研究会
交流服务中心

姓名：吴伟昭

性别：男

任职：特派联络员

任期：

编号：∅∅195020

有效期自95年5月至96年5月

As the former Accredited Man of the Exchange Service Centre "特派聯絡員" Master Wu was appointed to select national Qi Gong talents to join the Talent Bank and was considered the national treasurer "中國國寶". (Being a national treasurer meant that he was required to serve the country until his retirement.)

Wu also received the "Outstanding People of the 20th Century" Award from the World Organization of Natural Medicine in Nassau, Bahamas, June 2006.

5. MY VISIT TO CHINA

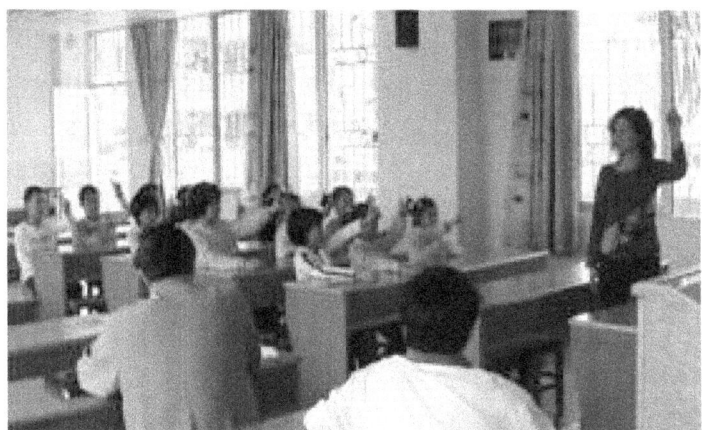

In 2006, I felt a need to return to China where Master Wu came from and also let his family know that thousands of people in North America and around the world are receiving the benefits of Wu's Qi Gong & Tai Chi® teachings. I took my new student, Erin Dixon, who is now a Qi Gong Instructor and Fa Qi Si (Qi healer).

I visited his hometown, a number of primary and secondary schools with Mrs. Wu in the Zhangchou cities through arrangements with the Board of Education.

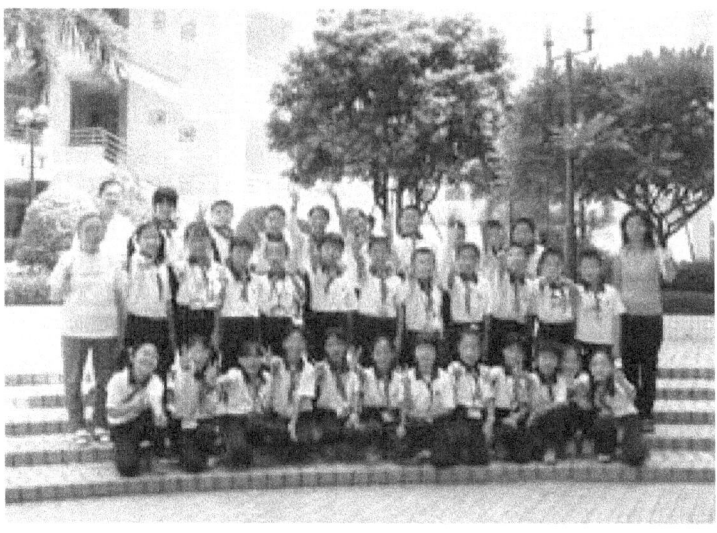

I was very impressed to know that children in the entire Chinese educational system practiced a series of eye exercises since Master Wu started the Wu's Eye Qi Gong® research. There were only a few students in each class that required eyeglasses. The teachers were a bit upset when they mentioned that there were some students who still needed to wear glasses. I did not know how to respond when they asked the question, "Why do western children with new technology need to wear eye glasses"?

While in school, all children went to the playground and exercised together, following an audio instruction amplified with music, which Master Wu designed for use every day at a specific time.

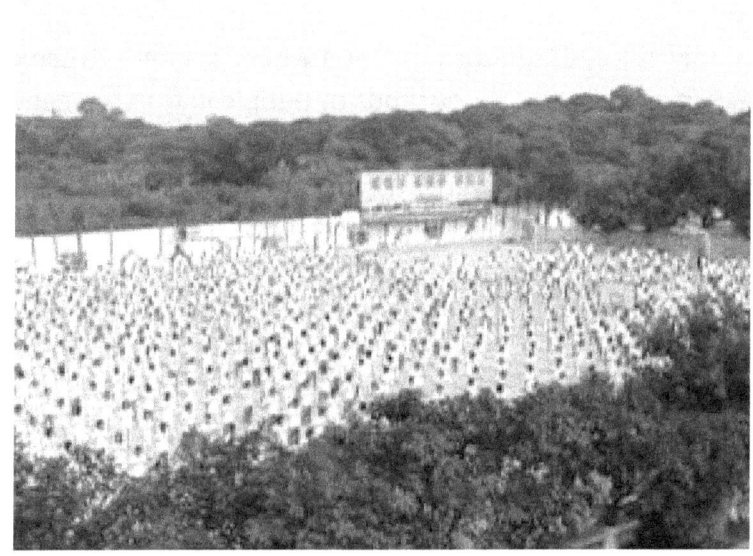

The children were humble and disciplined, and were very willing to learn. Children in residence usually hand -washed their clothes and hung them to dry in the high ceiling.

In parks, lots of people practiced all kinds of activities; for instance, ballroom dancing and singing. I had fun showing some of the teachers and children in a few Guangzhou City schools how to practice Qi Gong and showed them how to send Qi for self-healing.

Master Wu's colleagues, who worked with him, had great respect for him. Some of the comments were:

"He's a humble, kind and virtuous person with great leadership." "Today's Ghangzhou physical education system performs better than other cities, due to Wu's efforts of laying a solid foundation and his strategic planning."

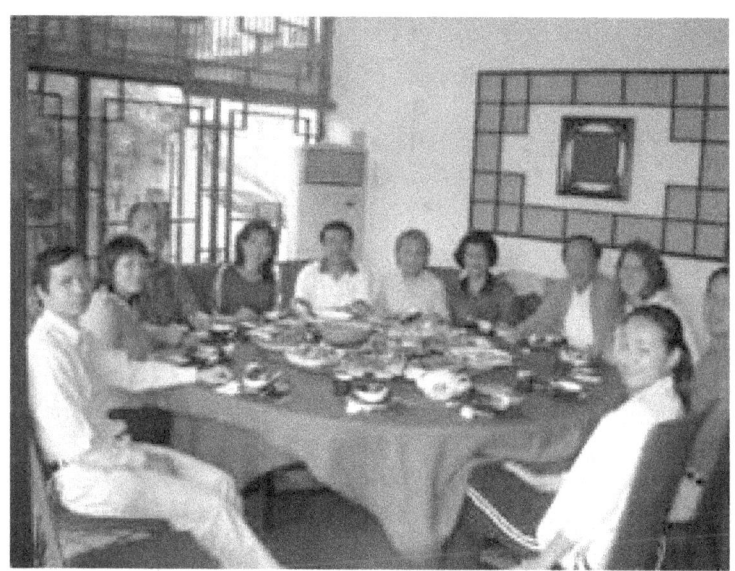

吳氏氣功格言

習歡云人少練功
撥骨坤筋敬眉綠
全身各脈盡放松
壽長省查清痰臍

總結多年吳氏功
功夫太極為基礎
一招一式循序煉
醒來壯陽先健腎
呼吸困難疏肺氣
舒張血管心次暢
遠年關節肌膚疹
癱瘓在床十叭載
八十老人穿針線
兩醫確診傳科學
陰陽雙修成絕技
吳氏氣功傳佳話
氣功不是萬能法

婦科卵巢水健腸功
淋池結節去乎遂
失眠夜尿剋果松
轉機全愈去穴功
近視煉眼去瞬朧
運壽惟怪盡去容
藏藏去妙在其中
有痛卽城未顯～
恒心鍛煉百歲功

A Conclusion of All the Years of Wu's Qi Gong Practice

Original Calligraphy and Poem written by Master Wu
Poem Edited by Teresa Yeung

Translation from Original Poem

Practice Kung Fu and Tai Chi to build a good Qi Gong foundation.

Practice Qi Gong with a scientific approach.

Practice Qi Gong to relieve pain, reduce inflammation and regulate the endocrine system.

Practice Qi Gong to improve blurry vision, myopia, and cataract. It is even possible to thread the eye of a needle at 80 years of age.

Practice Qi Gong to control our body and to produce more good cells.

Practice Qi Gong to clear old injuries and bruises.

Practice Kidney Qi Gong to improve reproductive system disorder, insomnia and night urination.

Practice Lung Qi Gong to improve breathing difficulties.

Practice Qi Gong Abdominal Qi Gong to improve women's system, live and gallbladder weaknesses.

Practice Qi Gong Qi Gong to make the heart and mind joyful and uplift the spirit.

Practice together with a man and woman to bring about more Qi.

Practice Qi Gong with faith, dedication and perseverance to achieve its greatest reward – a happy, long and healthy life!

6. WU'S HEALTH & FITNESS Qi GONG FORM

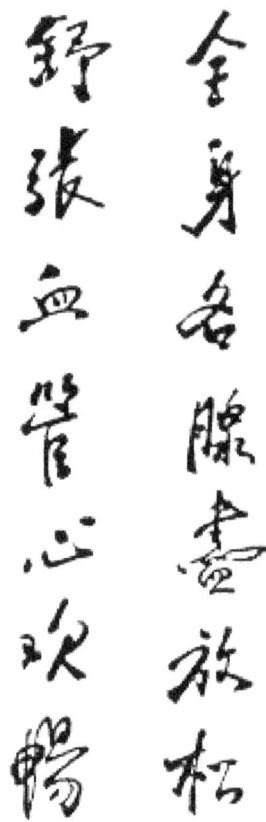

Completely relax all the glands in the whole body.
Relax and expand the blood vessels to improve heart functioning.

Wu's Health & Fitness Qi Gong™ is very beautiful and powerful 8-step Qi Gong form. It helps support your general health and recharge your vital life force energy. Many students with all kinds of health challenges find this form has very nice Qi and very healing. The Qi vibrates at a very high frequency, excellent for balancing our physical, emotional, mental and spiritual bodies. Traditional Qi Gong is long and difficult to understand and do. Some forms have no movements and others have a lot of movements. Some require a lot of standing and the postures can be difficult for people with physical challenges.

I was first introduced to Zhineng Qi Gong, commonly referred to as "Chi-lel" Qi Gong in North America. It is a long form that requires standing throughout the entire practice. I was trained as an instructor in this form by Master Wu. I discovered over time that our students love the form, but a lot of them found it to be time consuming to practice and often didn't receive the benefits it has to offer. I asked Master Wu to design a shorter form for North Americans who can practice for 15-20 minutes and still receive Qi quickly. Master Wu created an easy to do powerful Entry Level Qi Gong form in a few days. It's designed with the best intention to address the needs of North Americans who want to improve their health, circulation and immunity. This form has helped thousands of people internationally. It is. . .

- Is easy to do, remember and master
- Takes 5 to 15 minutes to practice
- Re-energizes and balances easily and quickly
- Safe to practice and flexible enough that you can stop the practice any time
- Awakens consciousness and develops self-healing abilities

The form consists of 8 steps:

Preparation

Relaxation

Abdominal Breathing

Open/Close Arms to Collect Qi

Up / Down Arms to Collect Qi

Project Qi

Circle Arms / Legs to Collect Qi

Collect Qi to finish

This Wu's Health & Fitness Qi Gong™ is very safe to practice and helps your general overall health and vitality. Many students with all kinds of health challenges find this form has powerful Qi and very healing. The Qi vibrates at a very high frequency, excellent for balancing your physical, emotional, mental and spiritual bodies.

Note: When practicing, there is no need to add other visualization techniques you have learned or read about from other teachings. When you are doing less, it can be like you are doing more.

It is most important to relax and loosen up the body as much as you can.

Step 1 - Preparation

Position: Sit about a 1/3 off a chair, enough to comfortably separate your legs shoulder-width apart and parallel to each other with palms facing up rest your hands on your legs near to your knees.

Head leveled, but with chin slightly tucked in; your back and chest straight, not rigid but relaxed. Rest your tongue near the palate.

Eyes are focused straight ahead, but slightly closed and lowered.

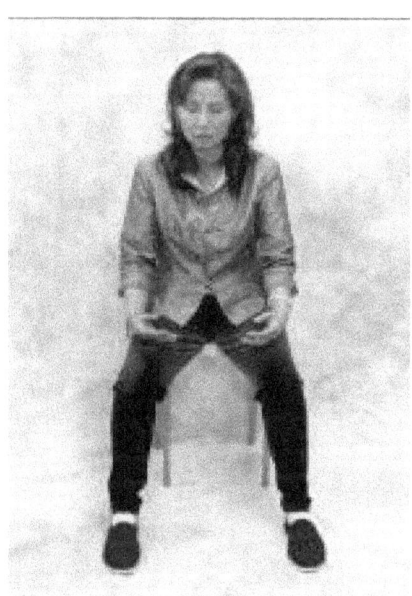

Step 2 - Relaxation

Relax each part of the body while breathing through your nose comfortably.

When inhaling, make the sound "soong" (soong means relax in Chinese). On the exhalation, repeat "soong" again.

Start with the head, neck, shoulder, chest, and then your abdomen, back, arms, hands, fingers, legs, feet and toes; breathe in and out for each part of the body.

Relax the whole body from head to toe. Repeat 3 times.

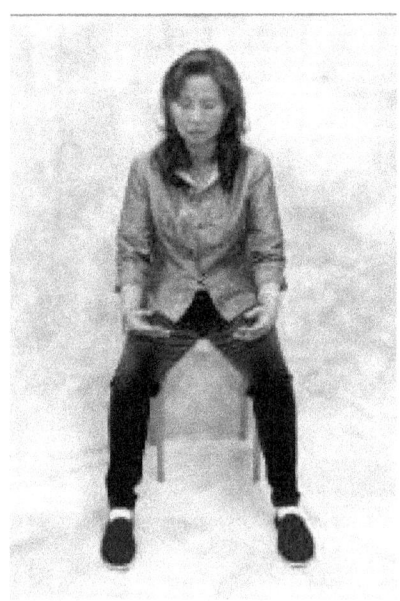

Step 3 - Abdominal Breathing

Position: Sitting or lying down, overlap your hands on the navel (ladies: right hand under the left; men: left hand under right hand).

Exercise:

Inhale and allow the abdomen to rise 70-to-80 percent. Exhale 100 percent all the way down to the lower abdomen. As you are inhaling, count: 1, 2, 3...to 7. On the exhale count: 1, 2, 3...to 10.

Note: For the first week, practice for 5 minutes and then slowly increase to 20 minutes.

These movements help to massage the organs. It's not necessary to focus intently on the breathing to the abdomen, which some teachings advise people to do. Keeping it simple is the best.

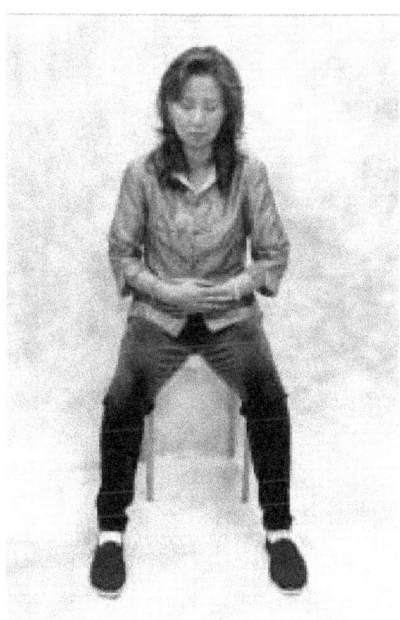

Step 4 - Open/Close Arm to Collect Qi

Position: Place hands in front of navel, palm facing palm.

Exercise:

As you inhale, open your hand "nose width" apart (about one inch) then open your hands to "face width" (about 6 inches).

Exhale, closing your hands to nose width. Repeat 9 times.

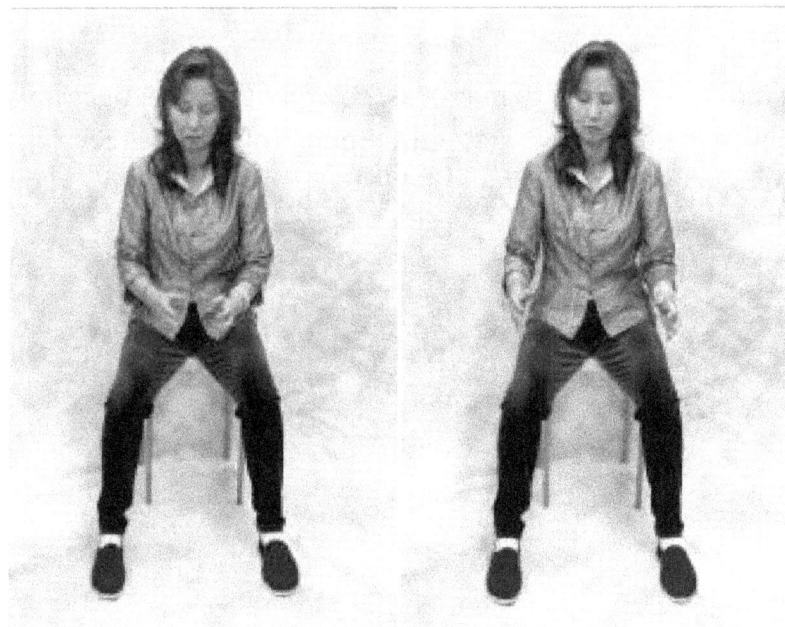

- Inhale, opening hands from face to shoulder width.
- Exhale, closing hands from shoulder to face width. Repeat 9 times.
- Inhale, opening hands from face to shoulder width. Hold your breath quickly and move hands lightly 3 times.
- Exhale, closing hands from shoulder to face width while moving arms lightly 3 times and exhaling the air completely. Repeat 9 times.

Pureland Qi Gong®
Wu's Hunyuan Gong®

Collect your Qi and the Qi from a Master, and unite as one energy.

Use your imagination and think of a lot of energy coming to you from the universe, arriving in your hands.

Take an experimental attitude.

You may feel warm and tingling sensations or even a magnetic pulse when doing these movements.

This new energy can be very powerful.

The feeling will increase with continual practicing.

Keep practicing best each day.

NOTE:

Keeping the Qi Gong practice simple is magical

When we keep the movements simple, we have more time to focus on collecting and moving the Qi thus giving more results.

Step 5 - Up/Down Arms to Collect Qi

Position: Move your left leg slightly back and stand up, place your legs shoulder width apart; toes pointing inward, center your weight.

Round your arms and position them about navel height, fingers pointing to each other. Slightly bend your knees hold abdomen and lift anus.

Exercise:

Palms up you raise your arms while inhaling to chin height and visualize collecting Qi from earth. Turn your hands - palms down – and exhale as you lower them to your navel. Visualize collecting Qi from the sky. Repeat 3 times.

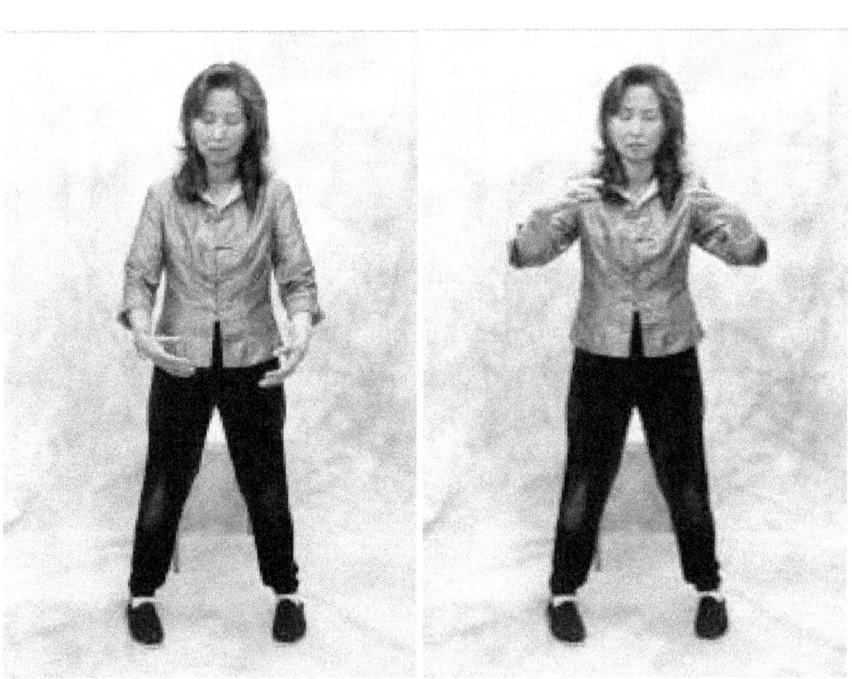

Step 6 - Project Qi

Inhaling softly, move your arms to cover the lower abdominal area and visualize sending "Qi" to the lower body. Continuing to inhale, raise your arms to chin height, hold your breath quickly and lightly and move your arms to visualize sending "Qi" to your upper body, including your head, neck, shoulders and chest. Turn palms down, exhale slowly and lower arms to navel height. Repeat 9 times.

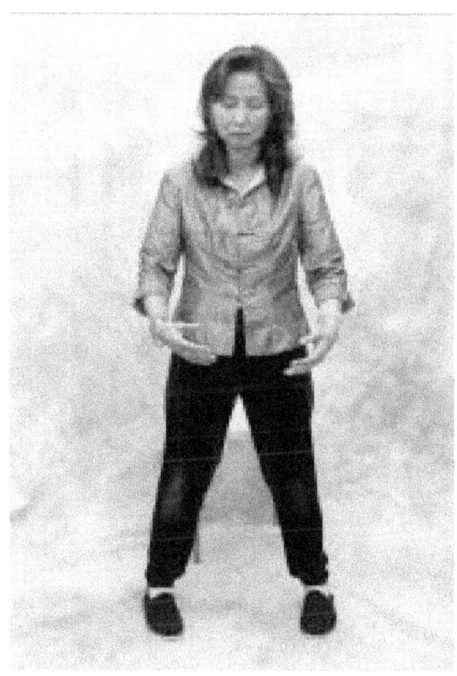

Note: Intention is very powerful. Visualize sending good thoughts and Qi healing to help you.

Step 7 - Circle Arms / Legs to Collect Qi

Position: Place your arms to the side of your legs, bend the knees slightly; turn palms down and leveled to the floor; fingers pointing straight.

Inward Turn

Bring arms forward to the front and center of the body. Inhale and bring arms toward your body, moving both arms at the same time.

When your hands are getting close to the body, exhale and separate them, circling out to the sides. Your knees move as your hands move. Your legs follow your hands' direction. Your eyes are half-closed, watching your hands. Repeat 1, 2 to 9 times.

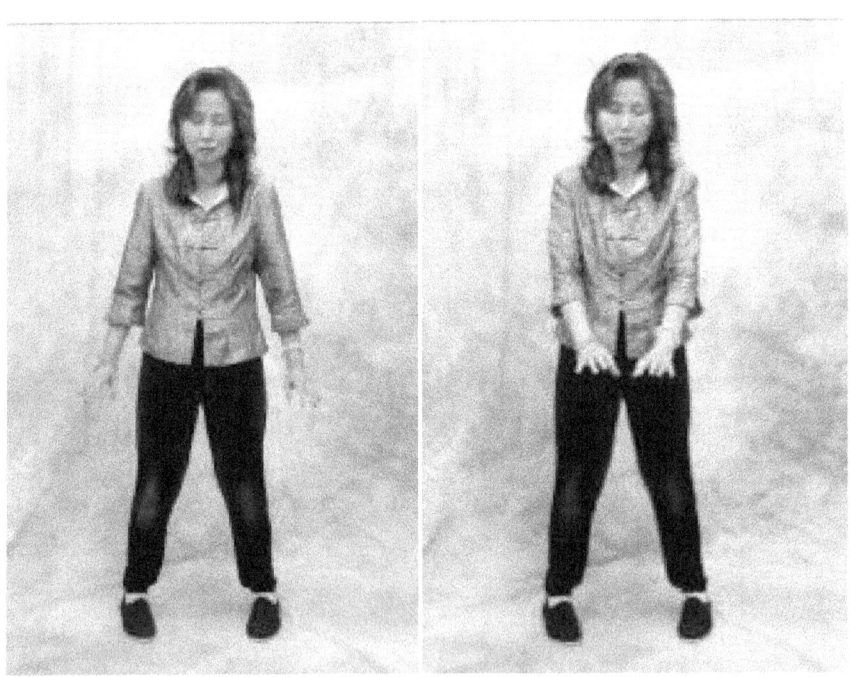

Outward Turn

Have your hands to the sides of the body, palm level to the floor.

Inhale. Bring hands from your sides towards the center body. When your hands get close to the body, circle and move hands out away from the body (the action is similar to swimming; knees moves as hands move; legs follow hands)

Exhale. Separate your hands out to the sides of body and position to the sides of body again. Repeat 1, 2 to 9 times.

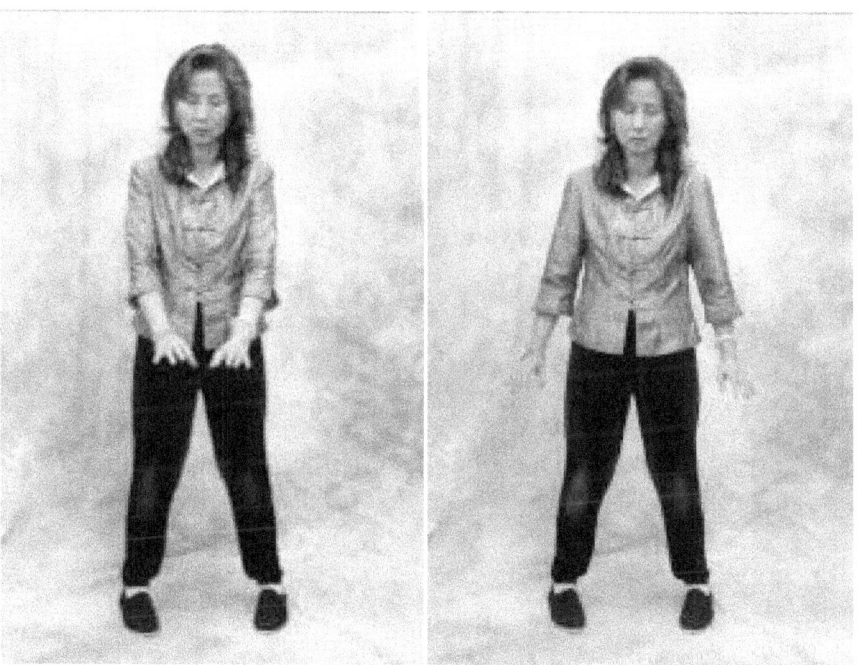

Note: It may feel a little awkward and uncomfortable doing these movements in the beginning, but they are very good for joint issues. They also gently tone the legs for longevity and work on all the joints in the body. If you are feel uncomfortable at first, do less number of times when doing the repeats.

Step 8 - Collect Qi to Finish

To collect "Qi" open your arms out then rest hands on navel. (Ladies: right hand over left. Men: left hand over right). Straighten your legs and bring them together.

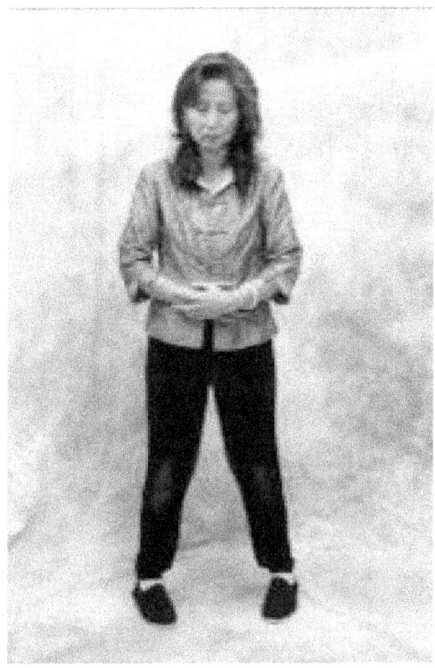

Turn hands in circular movements (9 times) Left hand: small to big circles, then right side: big circles to small.

Rub your hands together hard (9 times)

Put them over your face. Breathe in, wipe over face from side-to-side and toward the back, Breathe out (6 times)

Bend your fingers. Breathe in and brush back from your eyebrows to the back of head. Breathe out (3 times)

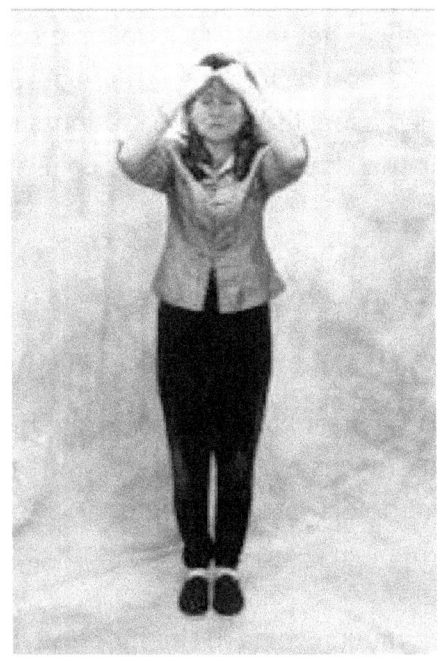

Collect "Qi" at the navel, relax and repeat "soong" from head to toe (3 times).

REMEMBER! I've provided 10 Do's and Don'ts for practicing Qi Gong to ensure you receive the most out of and enjoy your practice. I also invite you to use a journal to set goals or an intention for what you hope to get out of your practice. At the back of the book, I've provided pages you can use as a guideline.

In order to experience the full benefits, you must practice every day – twice is ideal; once is the minimum.

FREE

Grandmaster Wu's classic Qi Gong is shared on the home page of

PurelandQiGong.com

10 WAYS TO ACQUIRE MORE QI IN YOUR PRACTICE

1. The fastest way to get more Qi is to have someone give it to you. If your teacher can send Qi when you are practicing, that will be the most ideal. For this reason, I send Qi to students extensively in every class I teach to enhance their ability to feel, collect Qi and balance.

2. Each Qi Gong form has its use and purpose. Wu's Health & Fitness Qi Gong™ helps you feel Qi and gives results quickly and easily. The energy vibrates at a very high frequency. After a couple months, it is beneficial to learn a new Qi Gong form, for example, Wu's Eye Qi Gong™ or Anti-Cancer Longevity Qi Gong, because that will improve your Qi in other ways. You can interchange the forms and alternate them. For example, more Qi Gong one day and less on another. When you make time, you can have a very good practice.

3. Practice Qi Gong first thing in the morning. If the weather is good, practice in front of an evergreen, because it has great Qi. If you can, practicing Qi Gong twice a day is ideal - once a day should be the minimum. We have to eat each day, don't we? When you are traveling, find a place where you can practice Qi Gong there too.

4. If you are learning from a book, remember to relax as much as you can during the practice. Do not try to be too critical of yourself and worry if you are doing things right, or if the form is not correct, because this is not being relaxed. Visualization is important, but being concerned if you can't visualize is not good. Using a Qi Gong DVD, video or practicing with a teacher in person, on the phone or Skype is good choices.

5. Practice Qi Gong in groups to enjoy the group's energy. However, if you feel uncomfortable with others, it's fine to trust your feelings and practice on your own. Follow a Qi Gong DVD or video for a while instead. We have very good online programs for you too.

6. Set an intention to practice for 100 days. If the Qi Gong form that you are doing is not giving you any benefits within 100 days, it's best to examine how you are practicing it and find a teacher to properly teach you. Or, practice a different form. A good Qi Gong practice provides results fairly quickly. In our Pureland Qi Gong® system, students feel some results even in the first class.

7. Balance your emotions and release worries and resentments. Emotions burn a lot of Qi and it is not worth yelling or scolding people. Love yourself and forgive those who hurt you.

8. Eat healthy foods, drink plenty of water and sleep early. However, when you drink water, it's best to drink it during the day instead of the evenings to avoid stressing your kidneys.

9. Buy symbolic Qi Gong items to wear, for example, a Qi Gong T-shirt with a Qi Gong Master's writing on it or jade stones that have been blessed with Qi.

10. Find our Fa Chi Si (Qi healer) or Qi Gong master to open your flow of Qi in the body. It's like opening up the chakras in Reiki. This helps the flow of energy to move freely, giving better results faster.

10 THINGS TO AVOID WHEN PRACTICING QI GONG

1. When I started to do Qi Gong, I asked my teacher, Master Wu, if I should find books on Qi Gong and read. His answer was: "It's better not do any reading, because most books are confusing and hard to understand. Just practicing what I teach you is enough. After you practice Qi Gong for a few years, then you can buy books to read." I faithfully listened to my teacher and I never read any books until a few years later, then I understood what he meant. Different books teach different methods. Readers without discernment can become confused thinking what they should or shouldn't do in their practice. For this reason, I am writing a book that is appropriate for beginners to understand.

2. It's best to avoid telling skeptical people that you are practicing Qi Gong at the beginning until you have some results. Be aware that not everyone is interested in what you are doing. Most people like to tell others not to do something they do not understand rather than provide encouragement.

3. When you are first starting, it's best not to practice at least two hours before bedtime to avoid creating too much energy that makes you unable to sleep. Instead, find another activity like playing with your children, cleaning the house or taking a leisurely walk. After a couple months, you may find that you can practice before bedtime. The Wu's Eye Qi Gong®, other than improving vision, helps headaches, concentration and memory, and is a great tool to help you sleep soundly. If you wish, it's the best Qi Gong to do lying in bed.

4. Do not skip a day without practicing Qi Gong. Look at Qi like food for the body. Do you eat every day? How many times do you eat? So, you have the answer. If you find that Qi Gong is very energizing, you may find practicing once a day is sufficient until circumstances change. If you are a beginner, practicing for at least 15 minutes is sufficient.

5. Avoid negative thinking during your practice. Thoughts can be very powerful. Always think of positive outcomes.

6. Avoid eating "unhealthy food" when you practice Qi Gong. While you are practicing to make the Qi, your body needs to clear the toxins from unhealthy food. Continuing to eat unhealthy food is a waste of energy.

7. Avoid practicing Qi Gong that has no movements. As I mentioned before, it is referred as "Quiet Qi Gong". This is important especially for those whose minds tend to wander easily. My teacher told me that in China, this type of Qi Gong is not being promoted because of its adverse effects. I had a client come to our office who was very troubled by the involuntary movements this type of Qi Gong caused.

8. When you start to do Qi Gong, it's best to avoid incorporating other modalities at the same time. It will only confuse you and may not provide the results you were hoping for. For this reason, stick with your Qi Gong practice. After a few weeks and you have gained some results, then you can decide what to do next.

9. Each Qi Gong form is designed for a purpose and gives certain benefits. It's best not to "cut and paste" various Qi Gong forms together. It won't hurt you, but it will not give you the best flow of Qi energy. It's also good to mention who taught you the form of Qi Gong to honor your teacher.

10. Not all doctors like to know that their patients are doing Qi Gong. Please do not challenge them that you are using Qi Gong to self-heal and you no longer need your medicines. If you are on medications, please continue taking them while doing Qi Gong. As your health improves, check in with your doctor and follow their instructions to reduce the dosage if necessary

7. MY STORY

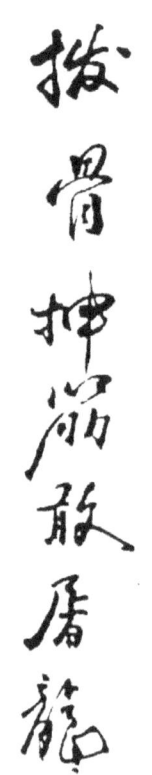

Pulling bones and stretching tendons conquer the dragon

I was born and grew up in Hong Kong with my parents, and nine brothers and sisters. There was only one washroom. My childhood was full of pressure with so many people in an apartment. Although very difficult, we received good education starting from studying in my mother's kindergarten school.

I spent my primary and second years at Maryknoll Convent School, which was one of the best schools in Hong Kong that taught classes primarily in English. The only class I could speak Chinese was in Chinese Language and History classes.

The integration of western medicine and Chinese culture were gradually becoming a popular method of healing. It became more convenient to swallow a pill or get an injection for an illness or disease rather than boil traditional herbs for well-being.

I was always energetic despite poor digestion and used to do competitive swimming and track. I specialized in the butterfly stroke and could easily swim a few hours each day. I also enjoyed the hurdles. After graduating from high school, my mother sent me and my sister to study Commerce Course to learn how to be an executive assistant or secretary. I was accepted in the best school, St. Paul's Convent School.

I never thought that I would get sick and continue to experience health issues thereafter. It began one night when I was 20. I woke up and felt that I needed to throw something out of my mouth. I went to the washroom and saw that there was blood. I threw up a few more times, and since I was not experiencing any pain, I quietly went back to sleep. I was taken to the hospital the next day. I was examined and diagnosed with a kind of lung disease: tuberculosis. Being contagious, I was quarantined, hospitalized for over a month and started taking daily needles for the next three months.

During that time, I could not immigrate with my family to Canada. They had to leave me behind until I got better. After the daily needles, I switched to taking medicines. Every morning for two years, I had to take the bus to the hospital on an empty stomach and receive 10 to 15 medicinal tablets in all sizes and colours, which caused discomfort and nausea. I remember there was always a nurse inspecting everyone leaving the room to make sure their medicines were swallowed.

I immigrated to Canada after a full recovery; however, my immune system was never the same as before. I got married and gave birth to three children. With the birth of my eldest daughter Rebecca, I had an epidural anaesthesia caesarean, because her head did not turn in the birth canal and it was not safe for a natural birth. There was a long line-up in the hospital and they kept postponing my surgery.

After the delivery, which happened at midnight, I had a fever and later my neck and back hurt terribly.

Thanks to the universe, I always met the right doctor for me. My sister referred me to Dr. Howard Vernon PhD and chiropractor; both my neck and back quickly improved. (I later found out that Dr. Vernon was a famous chiropractor. He was on the Faculty at the Canadian Memorial Chiropractic College (CMCC) for over 30 years and published the first outcome measure for assessing disability due to neck pain.) Coincidently, I was attracted to go into a Chinese herbal store and was inspired by a Traditional Chinese Medical Doctor, Dr. S. Y. Mak, who was also a surgeon in China, and started taking herbal remedies. (Dr. Mak was one of the doctors who championed legalizing acupuncture in Canada.)

Later, I had a miscarriage before carrying my second daughter and I was spotting blood. My experience told me to take herbal medicines immediately. I successfully gave birth to my next two children. From then on, I used more and more Chinese herbal formulas and continued adjustments on my spine with chiropractic work. I received help and experienced relief, but I felt too dependent on doctors. It was a frustrating time with my health and also that of my family's, because there were always one or two people sick in the household. When I was sick, I usually had a fever and felt dizzy and driving to the doctors was challenging.

I developed a problem with my right leg. If I walked in a shopping mall for a long period of time, I would limp at night and have to sleep through the discomfort. Today, I can walk for as long and as much as I need.
Since my 20's, I used to have a morning cough and constant phlegm in my throat. I was not able to speak for long without having to pause and catch my breath. Now, I don't cough anymore and my lungs are completely recovered. I can speak with strength and without pausing.

I used to wake up tired and could not leave the bed, but would not be able to asleep easily, because my mind was always busy thinking. There was also the occasional dizziness, which made me feel as though I had to throw up or I felt I would blackout. I needed to sit or lie down without moving for a few hours.

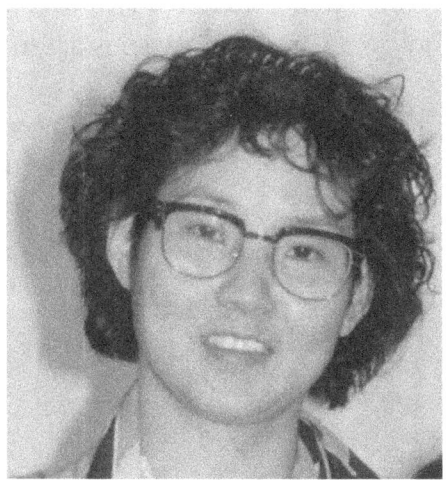

Photo of Master Teresa before practicing Qi Gong (1991)

I could not go outside into the hot sun for long or on a windy day, because I would develop a migraine or headache. My neck and lower back dislocated and I had to see a chiropractor for 11 years before doing Qi Gong. Since Qi Gong, my chiropractic adjustments held much better and slowly I needed less. I still go to a chiropractor or osteopath now for an adjustment, but only when I feel my alignment is off.

I had an allergy to cats. My eyes turned red and swollen along with itchiness, swollen throat and stuffy nose. I couldn't go anywhere that had a cat. After one year of Qi Gong, I was able to be around a cat for at least four hours before feeling the symptoms returning.

Now I'm able to be around them all the time even with all the hair flying around the room! My hay fever has gotten much better.

For some years, I asked people if it was hay fever season, because I wasn't feeling any of the symptoms. This was a real miracle. My Chinese herbal doctor, when doing pulse reading on my hand (Chinese traditional doctor diagnoses health by checking the Chi of the body), used to turn his head sideways, because I was so weak that he had a hard time connecting to my heart pulse. Now my pulse is strong.

I used to have many issues with my stomach: a lot of heartburn, aches, constipation, menstrual pain, diarrhea and gas. I had to carry pills for my heartburn; now I do not have any. I've learned to sit down and eat my meals and my stomach recovered. I do not need to carry pills with me.

After 10 years of herbal medicines and chiropractic work, my wish was finally answered in 1995. Now my health issues are in the past.

When The Student Is Ready, The Teacher Is Ready

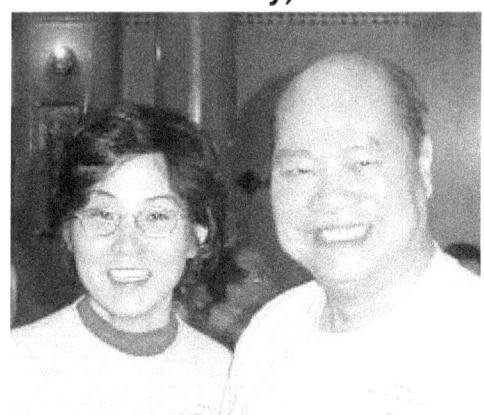

Photo of Master Teresa and Grandmaster Wu (2002)

One day in 1995, I received a call from a friend, telling me that his parents were immigrating to Canada from China soon. He was especially concerned about how his father would spend his time and the possibility of becoming bored after his arrival. He said his father was good in Qi Gong, Kung Fu and Western Fencing, and suggested that I find some friends and relatives to start learning Qi Gong with him. I gladly said "yes" and was really excited about the opportunity to meet my future teacher of Qi Gong. The next week, I met Mr. and Mrs. Wu at a shopping mall. I bought him a travelling Quick Snap camera as a gift and took our first photograph at the Mall. I'm really glad that I did that to commemorate our first meeting!

I remember during the first class with a few neighbours and relatives, Master Wu sent Qi out to us. Some people felt the Qi from Master Wu four-to-five feet away! I couldn't understand why others were feeling it and I wasn't. Was there really Qi being sent out or was it just people's imagination? I continued to practice twice a day. Finally, after about two weeks, I felt some warmth moving up my back and I was so excited that I called Master Wu and told him immediately.

I heard Master Wu talk about how Qi Gong can heal inflammation, injuries and different illnesses. I did not really believe it until one day our family hamster's leg turned red and swollen. I asked Master Wu if he could send some Qi to the hamster's leg to save us money on visiting the vet. He happily started healing in front of the children and me. In front of our eyes, we saw the swelling go down and the next day all the swelling was completely gone. This was the first time I understood that Qi could really assist healing.

Before meeting Master Wu, I spent some serious time studying Feng Shui, Chinese Astrology and Western Astrology with my Feng Shui teacher, Ivan Yip. I was inspired to learn from him after reading his interview in the *Toronto Star*. He's an amazing teacher and also a Forensic Scientist. This is a story I will always remember that impressed me:

One day, Master Yip and Master Wu met at my house. Master Yip was there to help me balance my house Feng Shui. Master Yip used a compass to measure the magnetic field of the rooms. Then, we went into one room that was not being used. Master Wu immediately said, "This room is not fit to sleep in." Later Master Yip confirmed he was right: the room's Qi was not appropriate for sleeping, as the magnetic field was really off. This impressed upon me how quickly someone could tell what's in front of you by his sensitivity to Qi. Now 17 years later, I am able to sense a place's Qi just like my teacher and I started offering Home Qi Blessings.

The interesting stories of Qi Gong always fascinated and convinced me that people should know about it, and provide a chance for them to decide if they want to practice it or not.

From then on, I continued practicing Qi Gong in my basement, parks and gardens with friends and family. At that time, I was 37; my eldest daughter was 10, second daughter, 5 and my son, 3. The children and family practiced with me, so I did not have to hire a babysitter.

Master Wu and I continued to learn from each other. I taught him English and driving and he taught me Qi Gong, Kung Fu and Tai Chi. On meeting more Canadians, Master Wu felt sorry for many people who were not aware that Qi Gong could help them with diseases that are common in society. Master Wu suggested that I do Qi Gong full time. I resigned from my full-time job, because I knew I could make Qi Gong successful, and I needed to put full focus on it. We started to do more in the Chinese communities.

Master Wu and I worked harmoniously together. I was the promoter and driver for all the years he was in Canada. At this point, it became apparent to Wu that I was the young baby an angel showed him in his dream who would be coming to him.

In January 1997, the Wu's Qi Gong & Tai Chi® Fitness Centre Inc. was incorporated. Dr. Ken Ng and his wife Emily introduced Qi Gong at the Total Health Centre and at the Federation of Chinese Canadians in Markham.

Besides being the principal student, I was also Wu's secretary, interpreter and travelling companion wherever the Qi lead us.

Our Qi Gong was shown on CBC Sports TV, the NewVR TV, and we were interviewed on Mojo Radio Am640, CBC News, Rogers TV and the Chinese, Western newspapers and health magazines. Communities opened their doors even wider as Qi Gong was introduced at York Central Hospital, South Eastern Asian Community Centre, Queen's Rehabilitation Centre, and helped raise funds for the seniors at the Chinese Richmond Hill Chinese Seniors Association.

For about 12 years, I translated all of Wu's teachings in English for classes and sitting in on one-on-one sessions. Watching Wu perform his healing was an amazing journey for me. It came to a point that whenever people asked him a question, I knew what his answer would be. As I became the scribe of his collective knowledge by translating into English these ancient teachings, I too became the teacher.

Later, by the invitation to the USA-based Supreme Science Centre Inc., we started spreading Qi Gong to Florida and later continued to other parts of the United States for more people to understand the teachings. With Master Wu's guidance, my teaching way in the classroom excelled, as well as in personal healings, promoting Qi Gong and Tai Chi throughout North America. I then became a teacher in the modality of Qi Gong, traditionally taught only by men.

In 2006, Master Wu crossed over into the spirit world peacefully, and in that sacred hour, the torch was passed on to me as his primary student in the traditional ways of Qi. After Master Wu's crossing, I took up the cause and continue the mission. I started to develop the teachings into a new level on how Qi Gong can balance the emotional bodies and how to use Qi Gong to develop spiritually. I continued my own exploration on how to connect the "unknown" mysteries of the universe with the use of the traditional knowledge that had been passed on to me. I received an "Award of Achievement" from the World Organization of Natural Medicine in 2006.

Keeping The Tradition Alive

I frequently asked myself, after Master Wu's crossing, who would be teaching this amazing art of Qi Gong if I died as I am the only student that Master Wu bestowed his teachings.

It became obvious to me the importance of having a broad base of instructors and healers for this amazing eastern physical and spiritual philosophy to move forward, so the Qi will continue after my crossing.

In 2007, I founded the Wu & Yeung® Qi Gong Wellness Institute, manifesting my vision to balance people's physical and emotional bodies. I continued to develop new Qi Gong techniques and explored the power of the mind, learning about and experimenting with changing belief systems and core emotional issues, using new methods to achieve Qi balance faster and easier.

I named my new teachings Master Teresa® Accelerated Chi Gong Techniques (A.C.T.) ™ and later Pureland Qi Gong®, based on this 5,000-year-old tradition. It expedites the method of collecting, making and cultivating the Qi energy. It contains the ancient secrets of masters hiding in the Chinese "secret tall mountains", including Wu's Hunyuan Gong® series.

The Institute is registered as an educational institution by the Minister of Human Resources and Skills Development Canada and qualified to train Qi Gong and Tai Chi instructors and professionals across Canada. Being authorized by the Government, students may be able to claim an education tax credit. Some programs are approved by NCCAOM® (National Certification Commission for Acupuncture and Oriental Medicine).

In 2018, I received the award of Chi Gong Master Award from Local Experts Group, Canada.

In 2022, I was awarded Health Professional Award with 1632 votes among 112 nominees. I received the most votes of 1085 and won the Grand Prize Trophy for the year in the 3rd Annual Golden Gala Award of EZWay Broadcast TV, radios, podcast and magazines, California, USA. The Grand Prize was to be given 30 seconds commercial professional made for Hulu TV with 880K subscribers for one month.

I continue to develop new Qi Gong teachings and various certification programs to serve the needs of the world. During Covid, I taught 200 over free or by donations successfully brought my work online. Since, I have been training remote healers using Zoom to heal without boundaries and limits.

I share Qi Gong with no religious or political intent, opening the door to people from all cultures who want to understand the art of healing. Promoting Qi Gong helps me to feel rich in my heart and soul. I continue my journey by continuous learning, discovering and evolving. Now I am working on a Qi Gong Foundation so that more people can enjoy this marvelous way of natural healing.

Family Qi Gong Practice with Master Wu

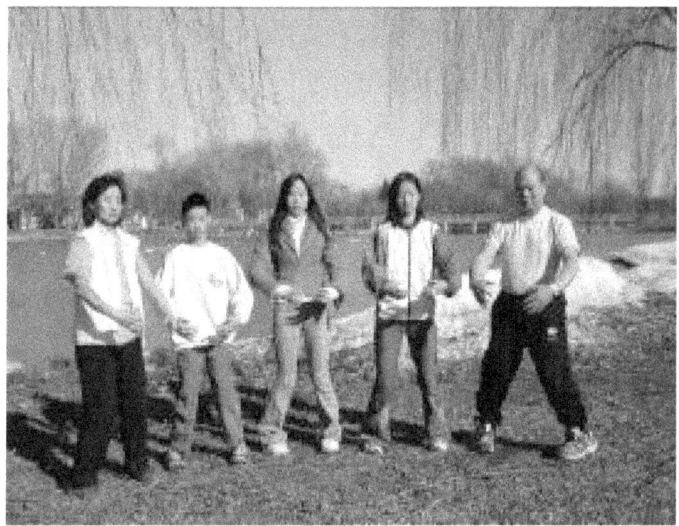

From left to right: me, Daniel, Rebecca, Jacqueline and Master Wu (2003)

My eldest daughter, Rebecca had asthma as a child and frequently got sick. She needed a puffer for breathing and wheezed at night. She could not do certain exercises or she started coughing immediately. After practicing Qi Gong for about a year her breathing improved, and she no longer needs a puffer or medications. Today, she is a visionary wedding and event planner with good health and can play as many sports as she wants.
http://www.RebeccaChan.ca

Jacqueline, my second daughter, loves to eat. When she was small, she had a constant tummy ache, especially after eating a bit more than usual. Before we went out for a big meal, I would instruct her to practice Qi Gong first so that she could eat as much as she wanted. She is a graduate of Psychology at York University and has a Masters from Ryerson University in Early Childhood

Studies. She is Qi Gong Instructor, Researcher, & Psycho-spiritual Therapist in Trainee. http://www.ChiwithJacqueiine.com

My son, Daniel at three years old still had a bedwetting problem. The doctors said there was no medicine for it and we will just have to see what happens. He started practicing Qi Gong to boost his kidney Qi and solved the problem quickly and easily. Today, my son excels in athletics, focusing on the hurdle. He has won many medals and was Senior Male Athlete of the Year for his high school. He was also inducted into the Hall of Fame on graduation. He ran for Canada's junior team in the 400m hurdles and is now studying at the University of Toronto.

It is important to note that Jacqueline and Daniel started their Qi Gong practice at a very young age and have maintained excellent vision thanks to Wu's Eye Qi Gong®.

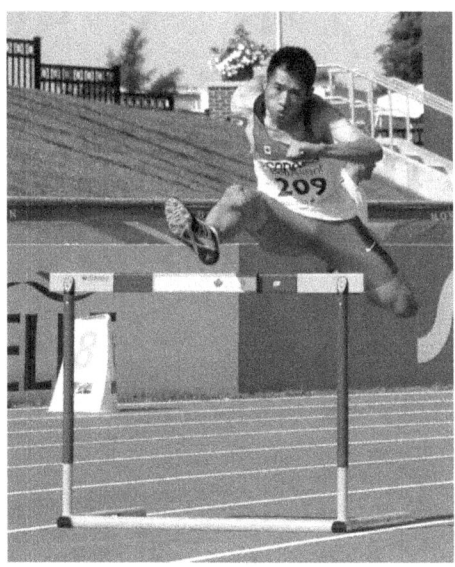

Daniel's athletic achievements:

- **July 2013** - Ranked 3rd place (51.76s) in Canada for personal best in men's 400m hurdles.
- **August 2013** – Double Gold Medalist: Men's 400m hurdles (52.11s) and 4 x 4 400m relay at Canada Summer Games (Sherbrooke, Que), representing Ontario.
- **2015** - Nominated Pan-Am Games Torch Bearer for City of Markham.

Since 2017, Daniel has served as an Athletics Coach for the University of Toronto Varsity Club, where he trained for most of his career.

Today, he is a Registered Massage Therapist focusing on athletes. Visit his website: http://danielChan.ca/

27 Years of Qi Gong

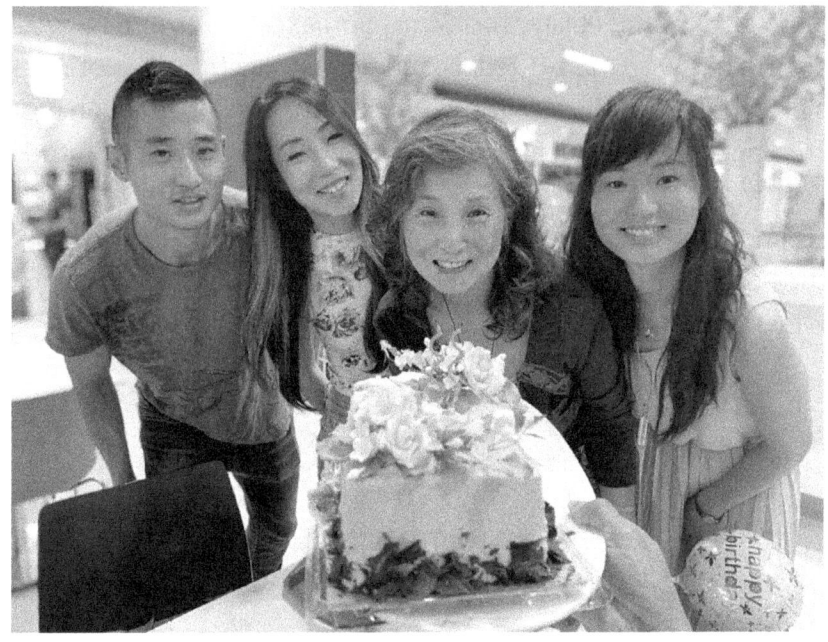

Photo: My 62th birthday (2019)
From left: Daniel, Rebecca, Master Teresaand Jacqueline

My Story:
https://youtu.be/pN5nTp-0Cg0

I'm very thankful to my mother, Master Teresa, for bringing us along as children to practice chi gong with her teacher, Grandmaster Wu. Without her as a pillar of wisdom and strength as a single mother, my two siblings and I wouldn't be balanced and joyful adults as we are today. We practiced chi gong as children and adolescents with my mother, Grandmaster Wu and the chi gong community. In 2019, I began teaching chi gong at The Hospital for Sick Children where I work, and I'm excited to see where this takes me. Chi gong for children and young adults is great! I'm working on my own book about these applications in greater detail. Stay tuned!

- **Jacqueline, Master Fa Chi Gong Instructor**

8. THE YEUNG FAMILY: GENERATIONS OF QI GONG

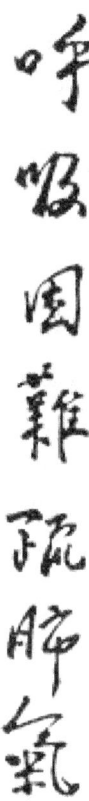

For breathing difficulties, circulate the Qi in the lungs.

Martin, My Brother

Martin had Irritable Bowel Syndrome (IBS) with terrible abdominal pain for over 25 years. He tried all kinds of western medicines to cope with the pain. The medicines helped for a while then ceased working. The dosages kept increasing to a point where the doctors became concerned about increasing them. After practicing Qi Gong for three months, the IBS disappeared. I remembered receiving a telephone call from him: he said, "I made it to North Carolina with no pain." It was a 10-hour bus trip. Since his IBS healed, he changed his job and became a renovator - a job he loved to do.

My Sister, Margaret and Brother Michael

Margaret, my eldest sister suffered from severe tendonitis, so much so she could not even hold a mug in her hand for any length of time. She tried many ways to heal without success. At that time, she already started preparing for long term disability, but recovered after a few months of Qi Gong.

Michael, who practiced Qi Gong, did not feel much Qi when he first started to practice. Over the years, he became so very busy with his work in IT, there was no spare time and he stopped practicing. After a couple of years, his stress level was so high that he began looking for help and tried Qi Gong again. He commented that: "Practicing Qi Gong definitely helps those in high stress jobs!"

Cecilia Ho, My Sister

Cecilia was 36 years old when she was diagnosed with metastatic breast cancer. It was a recurrence from initial Stage I breast cancer she had developed one-and-a-half years earlier. The cancer was very aggressive and her doctor told her it was incurable. Half of his patients at this stage did not live past four years. She began six cycles of chemotherapy, followed by radiation.

Below, in her own words, are her journal entries of her Qi Gong journey to help the challenges she faced during her chemo and treatments.

March 2000 - I developed Uveitis (eye inflammation of the iris) just before chemotherapy started. My vision was reduced to 20/50 from normal vision of 20/20, and I was very sensitive to light. Traditional steroid eye drops showed little improvements after three weeks. Then, I started seeing Master Wu for eye treatments and I also practiced the Eye Qi Gong twice daily. Meanwhile, I continued using the steroid eye drops. After eight weeks the inflammation was gone, but the ophthalmologist was unable to explain why the vision slightly improved to 20/30. The doctor stopped the steroid eye drops, hoping that the vision would eventually improve. I continued the Eye Qi Gong treatments and daily practice. My vision fully recovered to 20/20 within two weeks! This experience showed me that Qi Gong helped bring my vision back when western medicine could not offer any more help.

April 2000 – After the second cycle of chemotherapy, I developed an acute breakout of acne all over my scalp. This is quite unusual and may have been caused by the use of an anti-nausea drug. After two daily treatments by Master Wu, the acne shrunk significantly and eventually cleared up within a week.

May 2000 – By this time, my stomach became very upset and I constantly felt nauseated from the chemotherapy. Master Wu's touch treatment on my stomach one particular day brought an immediate rush of the chills from my stomach up to my shoulders and out through my hands. This was the most significant Qi Gong sensation I had encountered during the past three months. My stomach upset gradually improved over the next several weeks.

June 2000 – I felt some discomfort and pain in my lower left lung, while practicing Qi Gong. My doctor confirmed that I have bilateral pulmonary embolism (blood clots in the lungs). It is not uncommon to develop embolism with cancer. However, the doctors were a bit surprised that I was able to detect it without ending up in an emergency room. I was quite certain that the continuing practice of Qi Gong helped me to better detect abnormalities before it was too late.

August 2000 – I finished all my chemotherapy and will begin radiation next month. All along, my complexion looked well and I had a good appetite and ate well, despite the nausea. I did not lose my taste buds, which is a common chemo side effect. I feel and look much better than the average chemo patient, despite the fact that I had several complications. I believe this had to do with Qi Gong along with a change in lifestyle and eating healthy foods. I hope continuing my Qi Gong practice will help keep my disease at bay for as long as possible. Thank you, Master Wu. I hope you will continue your practice for as long as possible.

Cecilia

(Cecilia's story continued by Margaret)

June 2001 – Cecilia's cancer progressed and her doctors' prognosis was she only had two-to-four weeks left to live. There was an unexplored treatment of stem cell treatment, which may buy her another year of life. Instead, she chose palliative care and enjoyed the quality of her remaining time. It was at this time she decided to escalate her Qi sessions to help her with her journey. Cecilia was able to function normally, including her sight, while the cancer progressed in her brain. She spoke highly of Wu's Eye Qi Gong® and practiced it every day, three times a day. She should have been blind by then, but miraculously managed to maintain her sight. The day before she passed away, she was able to take her parents out for lunch. On October 26, 2001, Cecilia went into pain, shock, then comatose, and eventually died at 8pm that evening.

Cecilia was blessed with Qi that facilitated a peaceful passing. Her Qi remained in the room as she left her worn body behind.

My Father, Yue Kam

During my Qi Gong journey, my father, Yue Kam, has had a big influence on me and crossed at 96 years old in his sleep. His story is also interesting.

Yue Kam was born in Hong Kong, but later moved to Shanghai, China, to study. During the Second World War, it was not required of him to join the Army, because he was the only son in his family. However, he wanted to join the Chinese Army to protect the country. He believes as a man you should protect your family, and the best way is to protect your country first. When civil war started, Yue Kam and his wife (my mother) moved to Hong Kong for good. In 1979, he and his family immigrated to Canada.

In 1997, Yue Kam fainted and went to the hospital. His doctor told him that he had a blood disorder, because he did not have enough red blood hemoglobin and was transfused with four bags of blood. The doctor could not figure out why he was not making blood. After his discharge from the hospital, Yue Kam remembered practicing Qi Gong and Kung Fu when he was 11 years old. He started practicing Qi Gong again with Master Wu and his yearly physicals indicate his blood is fine.

In 1999, at 75 years old, Yue Kam was diagnosed with thyroid cancer on both sides of the neck. He had surgery and the whole thyroid was removed. He was given radioactive iodine after the surgery, and according to his memory, each iodine dosage equaled 10,000 volts of electricity! After swallowing two dosages, he was quarantined in his hospital room and not allowed to see anyone for three days. According to the doctor, most patients have five years of life after surgery with his kind of thyroid cancer, which means only 25 percent live past five years. Dad continued faithfully to practice Qi Gong and has never stopped practicing. Yue Kam is a 13-year thyroid cancer survivor.

In 2003, Yue Kam and his wife were driving back to Toronto from USA. It was a two-road highway; however, he started to see only one road. He knew that his eyes had a problem and stopped driving immediately. When he returned to Toronto, he could not get an immediate appointment and had to wait until 2004! He was diagnosed with severe glaucoma. Dad stopped driving completely. There is no cure for his type of glaucoma.

One day, Yue Kam was walking in the Mall and suddenly he couldn't see; everything became black. He was diagnosed with an eye stroke. The doctor said that in the future, he will have lots of pain, the kind of pain that's worse than cancer pain. He was also told that laser treatments would not cure him, but could help with the pain. Dad received eight laser treatments to kill the optic nerve so that it would never give him that kind of pain.

Yue Kam also developed cataracts, but could not have surgery because of the glaucoma. He continues to practice Qi Gong and receive Qi Gong healing from me. Although his vision cannot be completely recovered, he is able to maintain some vision to this day, which is a miracle. A lot of people have lost their vision completely with his kind of condition. He crossed at 96 during Covid peacefully in his sleep.

Yue Kam's Daily Qi Gong Practice

Wake in the morning and practices Qi Gong for 25 minutes
Drinks four cups of water
Has a bowel movement
Takes the medicines he has to take
Goes back to sleep, if he is tired

Yue Kam was Roman Catholic, and he liked to explain his philosophy to people who believe in God:

If you believe in God, then you can understand that evil spirit is also being created by God. Everything is from God. God is everywhere! Even in the washroom. Qi Gong is not evil. When you practice Qi Gong, you do not pray to anyone.

Yue Kam also spent a lot of time in Bible study. He showed us a thick old Bible that has research studies printed from 1968 in Hong Kong. He said, "It's fascinating to find out that when Moses was given the Ten Commandments, at about the same time as the Chau Dynasty in China."

In the Chau Dynasty, China had a few very famous philosophers: K'ung-fu-tzu and Confucius (founder of Confucianism, Lao Tzu or Lao Zi 老子 (founder of Taoism), Zhuangzi 莊子. Their great knowledge, wisdom and philosophies continue to influence China and the world still today.

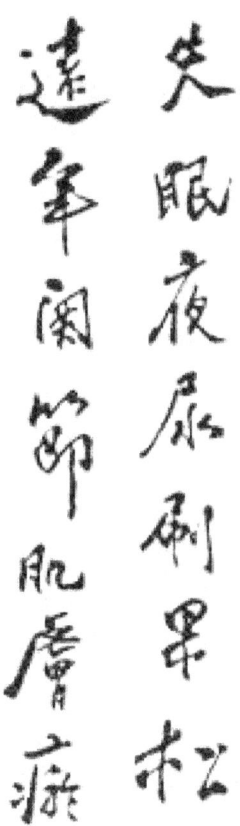

In the aged with arthritis, skin bruises, insomnia and night urination,
it's important to train the Qi of the pineal gland.

My Mother, Mary

My mom, Mary, suffered severe rheumatoid arthritis and her fingers and toes were all bent, crooked, swollen and overlapped. Qi Gong had helped her regain some mobility for her thumbs to bend and she could raise her arms higher. She had prescribed painkillers.

Over the years, mom Mary fell down numerous times and was gradually losing her appetite: eating less, drinking less; it became less and less with each passing year. When she was aage 86, she was admitted to the hospital for malnutrition; all her joints were inflamed and hurt to the touch.

While in the hospital, she told me that she wanted to eat, but had trouble swallowing food. She picked up some food and put it into her mouth, but she couldn't swallow. For the first time, I realized what mom's real problem was. From that moment on, I started sending her Qi for hours each day for the next few days. She became extremely hungry and finally could swallow again. At the last few doctor's visits, the doctor was very pleased that all her joints were cooling down from being hot, which meant her arthritic joints were in remission.

My mom's story inspires me to tell children with senior parents to stop watching their parents get sick and feel stuck. Everyone can learn to send healing to those you love!

My mom was very proud of herself, even at 92 before she died, she never needed to pee on diaper. She did not need much pain killer and even ate ice-cream a couple hours before she crossed at peace.

9. QI GONG STORIES:
PERSONAL JOURNEYS OF SELF-HEALING

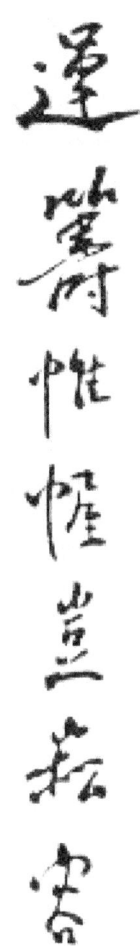

Qi Gong helps you relax and improve strategic planning.

Dr. Michael O'Daniel
(Warrenton, Virginia, USA)

I was a holistic chiropractor for 30 years. My practice included chiropractic, acupuncture, nutrition, applied kinesiology, quantum touch and massage. After taking Medical Qi Gong classes with Master Teresa®, I learned a powerful healing technique to add to my practice and also for my own health. When working with Master Teresa® I experienced mental as well as physical relaxation and a greater feeling of wellbeing and positive energy. My patients were responding very well and it was great to have this technique when other things weren't working. And I am now starting to use Qi Gong first for many conditions with the same good results. My vibration and healing power have increased and I enjoy my practice more.

Thank you, Master Teresa® for a new direction and a new life. Recently, I closed my holistic chiropractic practice and followed my passion for flying. I currently now teach powered paragliding.

Dr. Nicholas Ashfield - Chiropractor, Radionics Practitioner and Qi Energy Healer
(Toronto, Canada) www.torontohealingarts.ca

I am a long time chiropractor and director of Toronto Healing Arts Centre and my wife is a counselor. We went to see Master Teresa®, during a time of considerable stress in both our lives. I found her work wonderful.

Qi Gong is peaceful, calming and very nourishing for the nervous system and helps strengthen the endocrine glands. I highly recommend her services for one-on-one work, as well as taking classes to develop your wonderful growth of vital life force energy.

Dr. Ashfield is the founder of Toronto Healing Arts Centre, serving complementary and alternative therapy needs since 1983.

CLAIRVOYANCE / INTUITIVE

Deana Marie - Clairvoyant Medium
(Sedona, USA)

Master Teresa® is a true master in her field of martial art. I attended many of her Qi Gong classes. Her teaching and classes have brought a whole new meaning to my spiritual journey and life. I have taken what I have learned and applied it to my own teachings. It has grounded my work of healing on all levels. I don't know what to say except, "thank you" for what you have done for me and for all the wonderful people I work with. The journey has truly been priceless. I will continue my work with Master Teresa® for a very long time.

Elisabeth - Dowser, Qi Gong Instructor and Fa Qi Si

My experience with Qi Gong has been very positive since I was introduced to it two-and-a-half years ago at the Wu & Yeung Qi Gong Wellness Institute. I am now a firm believer of the practice of Qi Gong. I practice Qi Gong at least five times a week every morning before I go to work. I always practice Levels I and II, as well as Kidney Qi Gong. It helps me to stabilize my calmness and peace before I enter the rush hour subway each morning, followed by the demands of highly focused work and repeated interruptions of being in a busy, noisy, open office environment. On the days that I don't practice, I feel less in control of my sense of wellbeing.

I took Fa Qi with my "significant other". Fa Qi is a practice for sending Qi, mainly to heal others. It was really nice to do something meaningful together and to care for each other. We both really enjoyed receiving Qi from each other; being able to give Qi, and as a result, had more appreciation for each other.

After taking the courses of General Instructors Level I and Fa Qi Healing, I have begun to teach my co-workers during lunch, sometimes followed by giving them a Fa Qi session so that they understand how a Qi Gong practice will feel after they practice it every day over a period of time. Afterwards, they have all commented on how relaxed they feel and how they were able to cope much better during the rest of the day. They have even expressed the desire to learn more about Qi Gong. Level I is now an ongoing program at our Healthy Workplace Investment Committee's events.

On a personal level, before I began Qi Gong, the skin all over my hands was extremely cracked with eczema for quite a number of years. After learning Fa Qi Si, I began to use Fa Qi Si practice on my hands every morning and the eczema disappeared. I am a dowser and believe that using the computer which has electromagnetic radiation frequency (EMF) every day, full time for work, coupled with my sensitivity to energy, causes the eczema.

However, by sending Qi to my hands every day before work helps my hands stay healthy. When I don't do this, my hands begin to develop eczema again. Practicing Qi Gong is a great way to stabilize my energy before I dowse any type of energy, which may be detrimental to me.

Two weeks ago, I was sick with a flu virus and didn't feel well enough to go out and see a doctor. I called Master Teresa® to let her know that I couldn't teach a class for her that night. She sent me Qi to relieve the aches in my neck and I was able to walk out and meet her at a nearby intersection so that she could take me to get Chinese medicine for the flu.

"Feeling Joy As Pain Always Reduces With Qi Gong"

Laurie Huston - Intuitive Counselor and Radio Host
(Toronto, Canada) http://www.IntuitiveSoul.com

When Master Teresa® requested that I write a "success story" with my experience with Qi Gong, I was a little hesitant, as I am currently still recovering from two frozen shoulders. However, Qi sessions were instrumental during most of my painful period with this disease. I also know that Qi Gong is one of the only modalities that build energy within your body. Some may argue that yoga does this; however, what yoga does is keep your core flexible. This may result in allowing more energy into your body, by opening up your core and removing stuck energy. But it doesn't actually build any energy. It just releases and allows it to move more freely. Illness, pain, disease all have reasons to be in our lives. No matter what you "believed" happened that caused it, there will always be a mental, emotional, physical and/or spiritual cause associated with it. Typically, these causes are a result of outdated, unconscious beliefs we have held onto since childhood. This means you need to explore whatever is happening with a therapist or healer, etc., to uncover and heal the underlying reason. And we need to explore our motivation and resistance to healing also.

Master Teresa® was instrumental in building my Qi, which meant for a period of time, I would have no pain, during a time of 24/7 pain. Also, she addressed some of the emotional and physical causes to my frozen shoulders. For that I am truly grateful! We are blessed with such a wonderful teacher and healer as Master Teresa®!

To others out there who are seeking ways to better your life, I recommend beginning with the Introduction to Qi Gong courses that Master Teresa® offers. Then let your body/mind/spirit guide you in the direction most helpful for you. Thank you to all of the people who have been part of my Qi Gong journey.

ENERGY / VIBRATIONAL HEALING

Ed Dolezal
Founder, Universal Qi Gong & Tai Chi Institute in Palm Beach Gardens, Florida
Co-Founder Pureland International Qi Gong (Toronto, Canada)
Professional Member of the National Qi Gong Association
561-450-9630 www.UniversalQiGong.net

However you come to Qi Gong, welcome! Whether it's for curative, prophylactic or spiritual purposes, be prepared for powerful positive changes in your life.

Even though I was a Reiki Level 3 Practitioner, I was attracted to and learned Health and Fitness Qi Gong, as well as other forms. It resulted in the elimination of pharmaceuticals for my asthma and COPD condition. My pulmonologist confirms that it has been reversed.

I became a Fa Qi Si, Medical Qi Gong healer, and solely use this technique with clients now. Good outcomes are always reported by them.

Doris Markos - Reiki Practitioner, Qi Gong Instructor, Fa Qi Si and Hair Stylist (Stouffville, Canada)

As a Reiki practitioner, I found that Qi Gong creates a great amount of energy for healing. The ability to heal yourself and help teach others to heal themselves is very important. We all have the ability to self-heal, and Qi Gong gives us that opportunity. We are able to learn and use the techniques easily and very effectively. It will make the difference we all need in our lives. Thank you, Master Teresa®, for being a great healer, teacher and mentor to me and many others.

Learning Qi Gong will only be beneficial, if one consistently practices the form they learn. Master Teresa Yeung is a very good teacher and a medical intuitive. When the student is ready, the teacher will show up!

Jason Quitt – Energy Healer (Toronto, Canada)

I was introduced to Qi Gong in my early 20's to assist in building a foundation for my spiritual development. During that time in my life, I was going through a spiritual awakening and having many out-of-body experiences. I practiced Qi Gong as a method to heal and strengthen my energies so that I could go through these changes more gently. It took a good solid year of practice before I could feel energy in my hands and in my body. The more I practiced the more sensitive I became to understanding the energies of my body. As I practiced, I was drawn to different tools to strengthen and quicken this process. I started to integrate essential oils and crystals into my practice. This greatly amplified my abilities and Qi flow. Just by putting an essential oil on an acupuncture point or holding a crystal in my hand, took my practice to a whole other level of healing.

These methods led me on a very interesting journey into ancient systems of wisdom that can be utilized and practiced to awaken our hidden gifts and knowledge of who we really are as conscious beings. Qi Gong was the foundation of my growth; this is why I continue to teach these methods to my students today.

Julia A. – Usui Reiki Master and Fa Qi Si
(Toronto, Canada)

Master Teresa's Ancient Qi Gong "Fa Qi Si" Healing® is a wonderful healing system. I can actually feel a difference when adding the Qi Gong principles into Reiki treatment sessions. The result is wonderful. After each session, I apply Qi Gong and Reiki principles to clear my energy.

Qi Gong also helps me to focus better and easier. It has many wonderful techniques that help the Reiki practitioner to clear and improve her or his own energy, and transmit the life force energy easier and better during the treatment. It is also a very helpful way to enlightenment.

Thank you very much, Master Teresa® for bringing the Qi Gong practices to the world. More people are benefiting from them in ways to improve their lives: understand the meaning of events that happen, heal themselves and others, have better relationships, become more involved with physical, emotional and spiritual health for their own welfare and others, and for society as a whole. I definitely recommend Reiki practitioners to study Master Teresa's Qi Gong Fa Qi Si Program®.

Winnie Kosmo – Reiki Master and Qi Gong Instructor
(Toronto, Canada)

Before my journey brought me to Master Teresa® in 2009, I was already a Certified Level II Reiki Practitioner. In the last seven years of my life I began a deep search within, hoping to find a solution to heal my physical setbacks because it was emotionally draining me.

My personal journey has been one of asking the universe and praying for guidance to lead me to the right people, modalities and healing. Through Qi Gong I have found that balance, the healing it offers and amazing friendships it has created.

I also wanted to share this beautiful energy with other people, so I started the General Qi Gong Instructors - Level I Program in 2009. I found that once I got into the flow of this relaxing, healing energy, I felt much better, and since then, I was able to return back to work fulltime after a year-and-a-half hiatus.

Through Master Teresa's Qi Gong classes I am able to manage and maintain a healthy and happy lifestyle. In my personal opinion, Qi Gong energy creates healing, higher frequencies of thought and feelings, and generates unconditional love for all humanity to be influenced. All of this really resonates with me.

My personal goal is to share this simple tool and powerful energy with others through my Qi Gong Level I classes. Now, I am also a Reiki Master (Level III) and have worked on becoming a "Consciousness Shift Facilitator" as well.

How Can We Believe In Something That We Can't See?

What is the one thing you do every day without giving it much thought? Breathe! Inhaling and exhaling. You can't live without breathing. What exactly are you breathing - air or oxygen? The only way to see your breath is when it's cold. You see the hot vapour that interacts with the cold extremities. Normally when you are inhaling and exhaling, you do not see it coming in or out. You just know because your belly rises in and out.

It is through our breath that we connect with nature. Our intention is manifested through our breath. That is why when we are focused on something with great intent, our breathing becomes slower and more controlled. Now imagine holding that state of heightened awareness, but with everything around you. You will realize that you are connected to every living thing around you. It's like an invisible thread that connects you to your surroundings. It is through our thoughts that we are able to influence not just our bodies, but our immediate environment. We are all walking magicians, but the majority of us don't even realize it. How do we cultivate this? The answer is Qi Gong.

- **Hafeez Sumani, Master Fa Chi Gong Instructor Level 1**

HOMEOPATHY / NATUROPATH / NUTRITION

Bob – Nutritionist
(Toronto, Canada)

I had first stage Dupuytrens, inflammation of the tendon on the hand, which can be quite painful and difficult. Master Teresa® was the only therapist who relieved the pain after a few sessions. The condition has not progressed, which I am told is extremely rare. And I took one of her two-day introductory courses, which was really excellent!

Garry Tibbo – Self-Reliance Coach, Alternative Medicine & Qi Gong Instructor
(Toronto, Canada) http://www.garrytibbo.com

When you do proper energy work, and you are trained properly to understand its principles and how it really works, it's nothing but a benefit to you. I suffered from lots of digestive issues and I used natural medicines and plants to heal myself along with teas, but energy work was part of that.

When people test my blood or test me, they see that my circulation is far superior. I recently had my blood tested under a microscope, because I do blood analysis and the person told me automatically that if I keep doing what I was doing, I could live to 150 years. Well 90 percent of my blood cells had oxygen in them. Everybody in that same course, were far crenate or dying. They may have had one cell per slide that was alive, which tells me that doing energy work, practicing Qi Gong is very good for your body. I am living proof of it.

Garry Tibbo's *Free Living 101* – a six-disc set – shows a new way of living through finding natural wild plants as a food supply and healing the body.

Jeanette Sousa – Holistic Nutrition Practitioner
(Toronto, Canada)

I realized that my Qi was much depleted when my son was three years old, and like all mothers, caring for children and family, I was very stressed with the responsibilities of being a good mother, building my career and grieving the loss of two dear grandparents. Yet, I understood that being in charge of my own state and managing the normal stresses of everyday life is the key to any kind of success.

Learning Qi Gong has exceeded my expectations. It really changed my life and continues to do so as I grow and flow with my practice. Qi significantly helped me balance my emotions and release old ones and open up to more Qi. Every time I practice Qi Gong, it grounds and brings me into my body and helps me feel great. I love it so much that I became a Qi Gong instructor. I love sharing Qi Gong with my son, now nine, and we feel so good doing Qi together.

I am grateful to Master Teresa® and Grandmaster Wu for all their healing work. I feel truly blessed!

Josie Gintoli – Registered Homeopath, BIE Practitioner, Iridologist, Yoga & Qi Gong Instructor (Toronto, Canada)

When I first met Master Teresa® a few years ago at a Health Show, I was immediately drawn to the wonderful Qi energy. At that time, I was a Registered Homeopath and my focus was primarily on helping clients alleviate their symptoms arising from allergies. When I met Master Teresa®, I was feeling unbalanced and emotional in many facets of my life. She brought my attention to the fact that I needed to practice Qi Gong in order to ground myself physically, mentally and emotionally as a shield of protection before and after I saw clients, and the people in my life that triggered me emotionally. Master Teresa's Qi Gong techniques helped me to become more aware of energy flow, how to harness that energy and implement it into my daily life.

Since seeing Master Teresa®, I have obtained my Yoga Certification and Qi Gong Level I Certification through Wu and Yeung® Wellness Institute. Learning Qi Gong has also made a significant difference in the way that I teach yoga. Being aware of Qi has brought my yoga practice to a deeper level. Through the practice of Qi Gong I am more focused, patient and empowered in my work, relationships, and raising my two children. My eyes have been opened to a truly powerful yet simplistic way of healing on a deeper level, and my family and I have all benefited from this modality. Thank you so very much Master Teresa®, for sharing your wisdom and for your many healing sessions, which have helped me to continually grow. Thank you for introducing me to the beautiful, magical world of Qi. You are simply amazing!

Robert Posen – Naturopath and Pharmacist
(Toronto, Canada)

Any disease is an obstruction to flow. When you look at flow, it is always up and down; back and forth. If you take any Qi Gong practice, and you are still, your inside still starts to move and moves with the mind. The building of the mind and body makes for an exchange of chemicals; makes for an exchange of metabolites. It helps with digestions and it eases the mind of stress. It makes sense. It gives you sense and once you have sense, you have consciousness, and once we have consciousness, it leads us out of despair, which leads us out of depression and it leads us into a happier family life.

Ron Weston – Orthobionomist
(Toronto, Canada)

For many years, I have been teaching folks how to attain and maintain a higher level of physical and mental wellbeing by introducing them to the very basic and universal "Physiological Laws of Life".

These "Laws" focus on the following: our eating habits, physical exercises; contact of our bodies with the natural elements, such as light, air, sun, etc. and the development of emotional poise and positivity; rest and sleep, and occasionally true fasting.

With the practice of these "Laws", along with patience, I have witnessed changes in men, women and children of a very positive nature and this includes their pets, as well as numerous members of our more wild creatures, such as, for example, lions. Yes. . .really!

While on the topic of well-being, I wish to mention a very favourable experience I had while participating in one of Master Teresa's Qi Gong classes, not long ago. For several years I have been experiencing a strange discomfort in various sections of my chest, periodically. It was during my second session in her Qi Gong class that I felt a movement within my chest and presto the pain was gone! It has remained so ever since. The "physiological laws of life" are, indeed, universal.

Ron Weston is a renowned speaker who has been teaching internationally for 60 years on the secrets of successful living to universities, medical conferences and organizations.

MARTIAL ARTS THERAPIES

Bas Opdenkelder – Master Qi Gong Instructor
(Grimsby, Canada) https://www.facebook.com/indigoqigong/

I acquired an interest in martial arts and started taking classes in Holland at six years old. After instructions in Judo and Karate, I learned Pentjak Silat - a form of Chinese/Indonesian fighting art. During this time with Master Leonard of Silat Barongsai (1970 - 1980), I was introduced to Tai Chi and Qi Gong. When I came to Canada, I became a student of Grand Master Wei Zhao Wu. Master Wu had impeccable qualifications and a lifetime of experience in Qi Gong, Tai Chi and Wushu. Just before his passing, I completed my learning with him and received his General Instructors Certificate.

I continued to learn with Master Teresa Yeung of the Wu & Yeung Qi Gong Wellness Institute of which I am a General Senior Qi Gong Instructor. On top of regular workshops and weekly classes, I teach Qi Gong at Wellwood (helping people live well with cancer), a division of Henderson Hospital in Hamilton. Teaching Qi Gong to cancer patients is a life-changing experience. Qi Gong is not a practice you want to learn because it's "new" or "interesting", or because others are telling you to do so. It is a practice that should be taught by a qualified master (guru, teacher, sifu) so that you experience the benefits for YOU. One thing that strikes those who come to my Wellwood group for the first time is the amazing optimism that radiates from each and every member. When they start talking about where they came from, you fully understand why. Most were desperate and scared to death of being told their life expectancy was shortened. Among them, many suffered terribly with pain, vomiting, diarrhea, etc.

Teaching qigong in a positive way creates a relaxed atmosphere, which means a lot to newcomers, especially when they discover the number of people with conditions exactly like their own (or in some cases more severe than theirs), have felt so much better after learning easy to follow Qi Gong exercises. The practice of Qi Gong instantly picks them up.

My commitment to make a helpful difference in times of discomfort and emotional distress is an ongoing journey of deepening my understand of qigong as a powerful practice for health.

Cody Flying Eagle Templeton – Tai Chi and Qi Gong Instructor
(Sarasota, Florida) http://www.mindbodyfitnessforyou.com

When I was gathering Qi in Master Yeung's Sarasota workshop on my own, it felt like a trickle of water flowing from a slightly clogged shower head. However, once Master Yeung sent her Qi across the room, it was as though a fire hose flooded the room. I will sure be joining her instructor's program offered in November!"

Frank Zhou – Elite Personal Trainer
(Mississauga, Canada)

After just the first session of practicing Qi Gong you immediately feel calm and relaxed. As fitness professionals we are constantly giving energy to help others, whereby at the end of the day you are completely exhausted. Practicing Qi Gong helps to preserve your own Qi, re-energizes the body and also improves overall well-being.

Jason Schafer - Qi Gong, Yoga and Tai Chi Instructor
(Orlando, Florida)

I have experienced many healing responses from Master Teresa's teachings. Practicing in her presence has helped harmonize and build my energy. I feel vital and energized even if the work feels challenging, and I can sustain long periods of practice from the inspiration of our meetings. Her gift in communicating her work inspires me to practice more and build upon what I learn in her absence. I have seen evidence of her ability to send Qi to heal a small injury. For example, she moved her hand over a person's thumb and the area around the bruised tissue turned pink, and the thumb also enlarged to accommodate the new microcirculation to speed up the recovery process. This simple example is just one of many I have seen and also the easiest to verify.

The Heart Qi Gong she teaches is much more subtle and profound to describe than just sending Qi through a hand. My experience was of healing some mental/emotional tendencies, which were impeding my ability to be compassionate in certain relationships. I felt an energetic clearing of my heart chakra, which was quite beneficial to my sense of wellbeing. This was all preceded by a strong current of grounding energy which helped me to feel more emotionally stable. I am not swept away by any emotional surges anymore like I used to, and when I do feel some emotional energy expressing itself, I am comfortable with it.

I have been practicing Yoga and several other disciplines for over 10 years and have only been with the best qualified teachers in their respective fields. I am quite sensitive to the nuance and depth in teaching as I have been exposed to many different methods of giving and receiving energy. Master Teresa's programs are on par with anyone else I have studied with (this includes many well known figures), that also deliver good results in a very short time. I recommend her teachings to anyone who desire to take charge of their health, and also to anyone who has a yearning for a depth of Qi Gong knowledge.

Joh Friederich – Qi Gong and Tai Chi Instructor
(Burlington, Canada)

My background in martial arts goes back many years to the days when I practiced Tae Quan Do. Later I was drawn to Taijiquan and Qi Gong, including Medical Qi Gong. Some forty years ago, I was diagnosed with Type One diabetes and it has been under control ever since. What really helped me in this effort is my practice of Taijiquan, Qi Gong and Reiki. I am in better health now than I was twenty years ago. I studied with eminent masters like Sam Masich, Dr. Grand Master Yang Jwing Ming, Steve Higgins, Jill Heath and the International Institute of Medical Qi Gong. I have been teaching Taijiquan, Qi Gong and Therapeutic Qi Gong since 2000.

I was drawn to Master Teresa's Qi Gong Energy Plus® Workshop in Winona several years ago. Master Teresa's ability to project energy to the participants was an enlightening experience. My studies with her continued with Level I Health and Fitness Qi Gong Form - a very powerful healing tool for anyone. I was certified as an instructor and now teach it in several locations.

My own practice of Qi Gong, including the Health and Fitness Qi Gong form, helped me become aware of what is happening within my body, including sugar levels. Emotional and physical balance of Yin and Yang energies makes me healthier and better balanced all around. With my training, I am able to help my wife with healing and pain control before, during and after hip and knee replacement surgeries, to great effect.

My greatest pleasure in life is to teach others to heal themselves with Qi Gong. Healing others helps heal you.

Lee Anne Knight –Nia, Qi Gong, Yoga Instructor and Thai Massage Therapist
(Brampton, Canada) http://www.apathtoselfhealing.com

I was first introduced to Qi Gong through a Learning Annex class in 2003. After the class I knew I wanted to teach Qi Gong someday. It wouldn't be until 2008 when I had the urge to seek out a teacher for training. While flipping through Vitality Magazine, I saw an ad for training with Master Teresa® to become a Qi Gong Instructor. I immediately signed up to attend a free introduction, and soon after, I registered for the training to become a Level I General Qi Gong Instructor. I graduated in 2009.

In the four years of teaching and practicing Qi Gong, I have received many health benefits, including reduced stress, and a feeling of peace and wellbeing. When Master Teresa® offered the new Ancient "Fa Qi Si" Healing Program, learning how to heal others, I joined immediately with no hesitation and now I have completed Levels I to III. I am also certified as a General Qi Gong Instructor - Level II.

In early 2012, I finally felt it was the right time for me to quit my full time job in a law firm where I worked for 14-and-a-half years! I am so excited that I am working on building my career as a full time teacher and healer in Georgetown, Ontario.

Marcos Macau – Yoga and Qi Gong Instructor
(Miami, Florida)

Before learning Qi Gong, doing Yoga is more like doing a physical thing. Now after learning Qi Gong, learning what energy feels like, now moving the arm is not like before, it's like putting juice "energy" in your Yoga.

Saud Juman – Martial Arts Instructor and CEO
(Oakville, Canada) https://saudjuman.com/about/

I was the CEO of a software company in Richmond Hill, Ontario. I met Master Teresa® over 10 years ago when my wife, who is a reporter, featured her on one of her TV shows. My meeting with Master Teresa® was just a chance meeting. My wife wanted to thank her for being on her show and I tagged along for the ride. When I met Master Teresa®, I decided to try Qi Gong, because it aligned with my other martial arts practices. I took one of her courses.

When the time was right, I continued to practice Qi Gong, and Master Teresa® did different things to help me. Because of its benefits, I took my brother to have her help him because of a medical condition. He had a brain tumor that came out of nowhere. She was able to help and show him the root cause of some of his issues.

I also had a health issue and Master Teresa® did remote healing sessions with me. I had removed all of my wisdom teeth at once and was in tremendous pain. Her healing helped me tremendously. This incident was the catalyst to look into Qi Gong further, because I wanted to learn how to heal other people. I was involved with Taekwondo for 21 years, as well as cross-training in other martial arts. I invited Master Teresa® to do a Qi Gong seminar with my students.

I was Master Teresa's student informally for six years, but now fully a student with her for this past year. I had a small ligament tear and used Qi Gong to help with the healing. I went to an orthopedic surgeon and the problem was no longer there, and he encouraged me to continue. This incident gave me the impetus to continue and help other people.

Since my Qi Gong journey, I've had many experiences. When Master Teresa® was giving a session on healing without touch – using universal energy to heal others – she asked us to visualize the energy coming through our hands and to practice with someone who is closest to us. I began to feel the energy coming through my hands. I was able to see visuals associated with a given person's energy and related blockages.

Another time, I was vacationing in the Caribbean with my family and someone got sick. They asked me to take a look at their knee. After applying Qi to the area, the bite was gone and only a little hole was left. These experiences became interesting, because they are bringing me closer to myself. Not the small me, but a greater me who is the witness of what is going on - the unconditional Self – so to speak.

Through Master Teresa's guidance and lineage, I have been able to develop my ability to heal and work with energy far beyond what I had expected. I have started to do remote healing, emotional healing and have integrated it into the business world by starting to share with elite executives, CEOs and entrepreneurs.

Oprae Piao – Exercise Coach and Holistic Practitioner
(Toronto, Canada)

I find that practicing Qi Gong for as little as 10-15 minutes a day dramatically de-stresses the body, improves mental focus and increases my energy levels. Unlike a cardio or weight training exercise that breaks down tissues and uses up energy, Qi Gong is a kind of exercise that can rebuild tissues and restore energy.

Mark Brown – Qi Gong, Tai Chi, Energy Healer and Reflexologist
(Owen Sound, Canada)

Qi is the breath of life. Over the last 26 years, I studied various styles of Tai Chi, Yoga, Reiki, Energy Healing and Reflexology. Master Teresa's Qi Gong has been the catalyst to allow me to experience a deeper sense of peace, calm and better health in my life. The sense of peace in my daily Qi Gong practice carries over to the rest of my day. The deeper I get into my practice, the deeper that pool of peace is and the less impact the "waves" of every day challenges have on me. My overall health improved dramatically. My blood pressure reduced by 10-to-15 points on average and I have lost 15 pounds. I am currently enrolled in both the Fa Qi Practitioner and the General Qi Gong Instructor Programs. I am currently offering Qi Gong balancing sessions. My clients have shared that after a session they feel more positive, have lots of energy, their sleep has improved and they feel more whole and present.

By next spring, I will be offering Level I Qi Gong classes in both the Owen Sound and Kitchener-Waterloo areas. Thank you, Master Teresa®, for the gift of Qi Gong.

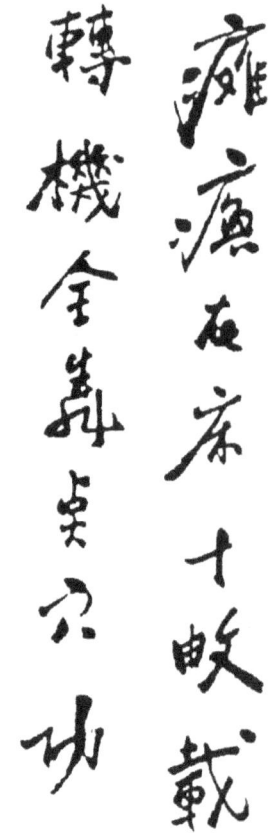

Integrating Qi with Acupressure healed a crippled person bedridden for 10 years.

HEALTHCARE AND MASSAGE THERAPIES

Steve Vetricek – Acupuncture Cranio-Sacral, Shiatsu Therapist and Fa Qi Si
(Mississauga, Canada)

Back in 2007, I was in search of needed pain relief. I started exploring new methods of treatment other than the standard western-based medicine protocols of medications and manual therapies. The conventional methods of taking medications were not as effective as they used to be, as my dose of medication needed to be increased over time to provide the same relief. That practice rendered me a medical addict and eventually I was required to seek healthier ways to live and acquire pain relief. I then tried several manual therapies, ranging from chiropractic to physiotherapy to massage therapy. The positive effects of chiropractic and massage therapies never seemed to last more than two-to-four days before the onset of pain again. The physiotherapy sessions helped me to get stronger with some more flexibility, but it never took the pain away. Needless to say, I became frustrated and felt hopeless.

In 2009, I found Master Teresa's website. After a few weeks of practice, I began to feel the presence of Qi and my pain significantly decreased enough so that my body would heal with passing time and with continued practice of Qi Gong. Having stopped the pain medication was impressive!

I had a few personal one-on-one sessions with Master Teresa were amazing. The peace and release I obtained was phenomenal, which I could not get from other healing modalities.

Once Master Teresa® offered the Ancient Fa Qi Healing Certificate program for Acupuncturists, I immediately wanted to join. On completion of the program, my Qi flows more than it ever has and I feel the Qi shielding me. I saw the Qi all around my hands and the feeling was just an incredible and joyous experience!

I am able to incorporate more Qi flow during an acupuncture session with a patient by building and sending some Qi to the acupoints that are needled, which helps to facilitate an improved outcome for the patient. By practicing Qi Gong daily, my health, clarity and awareness have improved, and most of all, my ability to help others has improved. I also want to thank again, the always delightful and somewhat mystical Master Teresa®, for slowly revealing the ancient secrets of Qi Gong.

Irene Vrbensky – Certified Reflexologist and Fa Chi Si
(Mississauga, Canada)

As a reflexologist, the practice of Qi Gong has increased my focus and also made me more aware of protecting my own energy. As a healer, Qi Gong has been wonderful as a self-healing method. I use to listen and balance my own organs and also improve my blood chemistry through deep breathing. It inspired me to learn Fa Qi with Master Teresa® and it is another alternative healing modality I will use it to benefit my current and new clients. Qi Gong is becoming well known and popular in the west, and I believe it will soon be a household word as it is in China.

Yumi - Shiatsu Therapist
(Mississauga, Canada)

As a therapist, I always wanted to know how to get energy back after doing Shiatsu on other people. Today, after this session with Master Teresa®, I feel very relaxed both mentally and physically. I felt the energy moving around inside me. It felt very warm - good experience. In my neck and shoulders the energy moved very well also.

TRADITIONAL MEDICINE

Dr. Joan Song-Nichols – Family Practice Physician
(Arizona, USA)

As a family practice physician and a student of Chinese medicine, I am very interested in and understand the importance of Qi Gong and its healing powers. I had the honor of attending seminars with both Grand Master Wu and Master Teresa® and experienced the power and wisdom of Qi Gong. Master Teresa® is a great teacher and healer and I am enriched from the experience of attending her seminars.

Dr. Douglas Nelson – Family Physician and Qi Gong Instructor
(Florida, USA)

I have been a student of Master Teresa Yeung for several years. I have taken a wide range of her courses and workshops, and recently graduated from the Level I Qi Gong Instructor's Program.

The training I have received from Master Teresa® has been extraordinary, and absolutely indispensable to my work and life. The benefits to my own health have been concrete and enduring. Through the practice of Health and Fitness Qi Gong, I am able to manage the stresses of running a busy practice more effectively and calmly. My energy level is very clearly higher, as well as more consistent throughout the day and week. My patients are benefiting from the Qi Gong exercises I teach them and many report reduced stress levels, improved blood pressure control and markedly reduced symptoms of anxiety and depression.

I particularly encourage other physicians to experience this remarkable healing discipline, which can improve their own wellbeing and performance, and transform the health of their patients. I'm sure that many professionals would quickly grasp the very practical benefits of Qi Gong, and see how it can be integrated into their professional practices.

I highly recommend any workshop offered by Master Teresa® to anyone seeking to maintain health, speedy recovery from physical conditions, or raise fitness and energy levels. Master Teresa® is a consummate professional, a gifted and caring instructor, and a true master of this powerful art.

PSYCHOTHERAPY / COUNSELING

Corinne Engel - Psychotherapist, Personal Development Facilitator, Published Author
(Toronto, Canada)

Qi Gong has been a healing methodology for my body, mind and spirit. Besides having a calming and balancing effect on me, I have experienced profound physical healing. One example is when I had a cyst in my cheek that had been there for 25 years. Through only three treatments with Master Teresa®, the cyst dissolved and disappeared. I was totally amazed at this result. I was astounded at the fact that this was even possible. It has been several years since those treatments and the cyst has never returned.

Emily - Clinical Psychologist
(Sarasota, Florida)

The partner's Qi Gong exercises in "Be Your Own Healer" workshop with Master Teresa® were a very powerful experience for me. I felt a wave of energy so strong that, for a moment, I thought a fan had been turned on. This practice has healing effects that I would like to see utilized within the health care community. I am looking forward to applying aspects of this practice with my patients, particularly those who suffer from depression and anxiety. Qi Gong appears to have great potential to soothe mental distress.

Rita Anderson – Counselor for Addictions and Qi Gong Instructor
(Toronto, Canada)

I read about Qi Gong and called a few places, but nobody called me back. So my friend and I went to one of these Whole Life Expos, and turned the corner and it was, Qi Gong. I went into the booth and Master Teresa® was showing how energy works and how you can make one hand longer than the other one. When I saw proof I was sold on it. At that time I was on crutches. I had injured my leg severely and had been on crutches already for about 11 months. I went to her workshop and I was able to leave the workshop without the crutches. Qi Gong is marvelous and it has helped me in many different areas. It's an amazing healing process. I am now in the Instructor Program.

Psychotherapist

I have been a therapist for nearly 25 years, beginning in 1988 as a Dance/Movement Therapist. Respect for the body's ways of communicating and healing are a passion of mine. When I obtained my graduate degree in Counseling Psychology, I accepted a job as a Clinical Coordinator for an agency that counsels people who have experienced sexual abuse. Over the years, this became very stressful and I eventually burned out. I suffered from various mental health issues, then left my job. I received therapy and medication, but I knew there must be something more. My husband introduced me to Master Teresa®, and we began taking some of her courses. We enrolled in the Fa Qi Program, which went for a period of about nine months. This was one of the most important things I have done, especially for my own self-healing, and also as a means of helping others.

Jacqueline Chan – Senior Qi Gong Instructor
MA, MPS Candidate (2022)
http://chiwithjacqueline.com/
(Toronto, Canada)

Practicing qigong has been a part of my life, since I was about 5 years old. It's taught me that energy is the basis of life. As an academically trained person in research and now, as a (budding) licensed psychotherapist, I'm excited about the benefits of qigong psycho-somatically. Qigong has benefits to the mind, body, and soul - and helps us build those neuroconnections between the mind, body, and heart. Lastly, teaching qigong is now an important part of my life and I'm excited to continue this mission! I'll be taking clients starting in 2024.

Julie Tirakian – Qi Gong Instructor
Julie.tirakian@gmail.com
(Michigan, USA)

I first heard about Qi Gong from a spiritual teacher. He told me that much energy was needed to make positive changes in my life, and that Qi Gong was the best way to balance and fortify the body with energy quickly. At that time, I purchased a Qi Gong video online and practiced frequently for a few months. Eventually, I became bored with the video and fell out of the habit of practicing.

Years later, I was troubled by arthritis pain, and someone suggested contacting Master Teresa for a personal session. The chi really helped, and I became interested in resuming my practice. I attended classes with Master Teresa, and I really loved the energy. I wanted to learn more, so I purchased the book, "Healing Life Force Energy", and began practicing on my own. At first, I didn't feel very successful. I had doubts that I was even doing it "right". One thing the book said was that it is important to practice consistently for 100 days before deciding about
whether to continue. I made the commitment to practice two times daily for 100 days, and my miracle began.

After just a few weeks, I felt more grounded, positive, centered and more peaceful. Things didn't seem to upset me as they had in the past. I literally forgot about my knee pain. Life just got…. better. I felt happier in general. Suffice it to say, I. Was. Hooked. I have practiced Qi Gong twice every day since.

I continue to learn with each practice. Today I am a certified Level 1 Qi Gong instructor, and I love what I do. I am currently working on Level 2, excited about what the future holds.

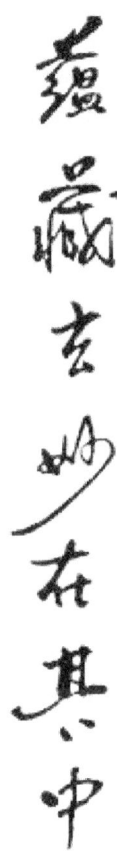

Great secrets, mysterious wisdom exists within the Qi Gong practice.

10. PERSONAL TRANSFORMATION IN ONE WEEK

Alex Drake
(Toronto Canada)

My mom has been diagnosed with breast cancer, and she has lots of pain. I wanted to help her. I found Master Teresa and have been working with her. I started to do the Fa Chi Online 2-Day Program to learn how to send chi to help my mother.

After a week of practicing it, I personally felt the difference in myself. I stopped drinking. I would usually spend $400 a month drinking with friends! I've become more aware, and feel a lot of energy and at peace. I feel that I can do something nice in this life by providing healing services to other people.

(* Whether it is over excess in alcohol or drugs, to support Alex's story, I have included a research article on external Qi Gong healing to reduce cocaine cravings: https://www.ncbi.nlm.nih.gov/pmc/articles/PMC3576894/)

11. OTHER PERSONAL STORIES

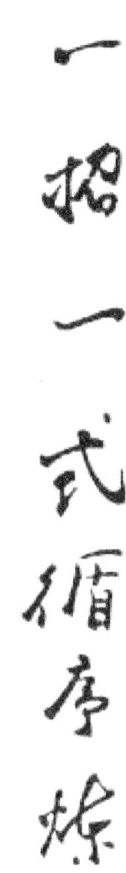

Practice each Qi Gong movement and style systematically.

Allergies

As our life force energy improves, it is common to naturally improve symptoms of allergies. All my life before practicing Qi Gong that I have severe allergies to cats. However after one year of practice, I can stay with cats for 4 hours. Now I have absolutely no issues with cats and can even enjoy having them around me.

Emily Ng

I met Master Wu when he first started his practice. I was pregnant with my third child and couldn't take any medications. I suffered from allergies really badly. I was coughing and sneezing and really suffering. Master Wu gave me Qi and showed me exercises to do. I was very calm when I had my baby and was out of bed and walking around the next day. Before, when I had my last two children, it took me a week before I could walk around and I had a lot of pain.

Inspiring Videos

Youtube.com/c/PurelandQiGong

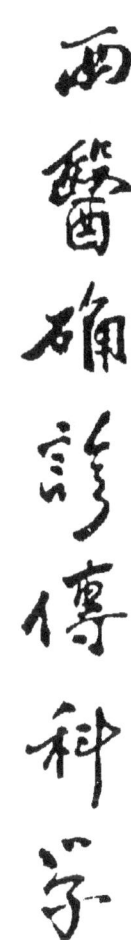

Western doctors perform scientific diagnoses.

Anterior Crucial Ligament

Gospodin Dimov
(Toronto, Ontario)

I was born and raised in Bulgaria. Soon after graduating from medical school, my wife and I immigrated to Canada. In the spring of 2009, while playing soccer, I tore a ligament in my right knee. The medical diagnosis was confirmed as a torn ACL (anterior crucial ligament), on the MRI. According to western medicine, a torn ACL can only get better with surgery. The orthopedic surgeon scheduled me for the operation. The wait for the operation was so long, I decided to explore other remedies. Going to Master Teresa® I was so surprised to hear that Qi Gong can actually help my situation. I joined the two-day Qi EnergyPlus® workshop and was fascinated with the feelings of Qi energy and the ACL pain actually lessoning in my first class. But I still had disbelief that it might be healing. It took me some time, but in the end I decided to give Qi Gong a chance to really work on my knee.

I visited Master Teresa® a couple times for private sessions and seriously started sending Qi to myself to assist with my recovery. In a couple of months I saw a significant difference and that made me postpone the operation. The knee now was 98/99 percent healthy and I was able to perform my daily activities without discomfort.

Because of my personal experience in my own health recovery, I am seriously thinking of learning and mastering Qi Gong, so I can be of help to many people. Thank you, Master Teresa®!

Gospodin's ebook: *The Great Integrity* discusses raising human consciousness through exploring ones sexual nature. It has just been published. ISBN:9781452573014

Bone Spurs

Richard Todd - Aerospace Scientist
(Cocoa, Florida)

The first thing I noticed about Master Teresa® was the brightness of the energy she radiates. Not literally bright, but the kind of energy that makes everyone present feel welcome, energized, uplifted and happy. While in session with Master Teresa® the energy in the room is palpable. She succeeds in getting everyone present to reach their own realization of the reality of Qi, by amplifying the natural flow of energy to the point that all can experience it. I have been the recipient of Master Teresa's energy healing for bone spurs in one foot. With one session, she set me on the road to recovery from an ailment that had been getting progressively worse. In a few weeks, I recovered to the point that I could actually forget about my feet while walking.

DeQuirvain's Tenosynovitis

David Duhaime – Fa Qi Si
(Toronto, Canada)

I was diagnosed with DeQuirvain's Tenosynovitis (a painful condition that affects the tendons on the thumb side of the wrist) in November 2009 and the recommendation put forth by my doctor was to go for physiotherapy. After five months of physiotherapy my pain did not decrease at all. Once I started Qi Gong treatments in April 2010, I noticed reduction in pain on the first day. By doing daily Health & Fitness Qi Gong, along with clearing emotional issues through Heart Qi Gong, I was able to return to my normal physical activity at the beginning of November (2010). Within six months, my wrist was completely healed.

Because I had achieved amazing healing results with Qi Gong, I decided to join the Fa Qi Si Program and learn to balance others who need help. I have a passion for helping people and assisting with their healing process. I felt it was important that people experience the same positive results that I achieved with Qi Gong. By learning Fa Qi Si I am now able to do so.

I suffered with terrible headaches for a couple of years and constantly needed to take painkillers every day so that I could function. As I was going through the Fa Qi Si Program, I learned how to aid my own recovery through deep work with my own energy, along with receiving Qi from my fellow classmates to help balance me.

On the last day of the Level III Fa Qi Si Program, I was able to connect with my inner self and asked that I no longer require taking painkillers. From that day forward I don't have headaches, and I have not taken painkillers. It's a miracle for me!

I look forward to my continuous journey working towards becoming a master of energy!

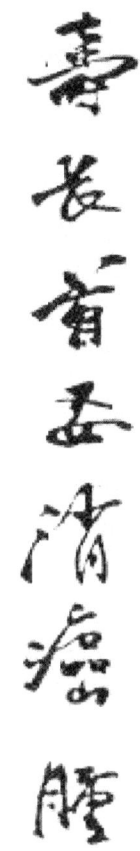

Clearing cancerous inflammation increases longevity.

Cancer (Cervical)

Christine A.
(Toronto, Canada)

In the spring of 2011, I was diagnosed with cancer. I was initially astounded to find out that the tumor was too large to remove surgically. The recommended treatment was radical radiation and chemotherapy.

A diagnosis of cancer brings about a lot of fear and panic to the patient. I did not want to decide on a treatment in that state of initial shock and fear. I was aware of a number of alternative treatments, including Qi Gong. Qi Gong greatly assisted me to stay calm and to check in with my body's energetic system to see what needed to be balanced. By practicing deep breathing every day, Qi Gong allowed me to strengthen my immune system and oxygenate my cells better, giving me time to heal. I chose to stop radiation after only a few sessions and forego chemotherapy altogether. My next MRI, which was done eight months after the diagnosis, showed an 85 percent reduction in the size of the tumor.

Cancer (Breast)

Jennifer Jo
(Toronto, Canada)

I was diagnosed with refractory breast cancer and had to undergo highly extensive radiation to my chest wall twice a day. The first week I was very tired, in pain and discomfort, due to the severe swelling of my auxiliary area. I had to take pain killers to sleep at night.

I then began daily therapy Qi Gong sessions, usually after my radiation treatments. I didn't have to take painkillers during the remainder of my radiation treatment. I felt so energized after receiving Qi that I was able to carry out my daily activities as usual.

I strongly recommend therapy sessions with Master Teresa® for anyone receiving chemo or radiation treatments for cancer.

Cancer (Breast)

Andrea Brown
(Toronto, Canada)

I was diagnosed with breast cancer and following the mastectomy, my right arm developed lymphedema (swelling in the arm). I started to do Qi Gong and healing sessions. The swellings came down and my hands began to look normal again, which never happened before. I had more energy and overall felt better.

Practicing Qi Gong is very good for people with breast cancer and I would like to improve my practice.

Cancer (Liver)

Mark
(Toronto, Canada)

Before I started practicing Qi Gong, I was lacking in energy and my complexion was pale. After about two weeks of Qi Gong, the colour returned to my face and hands.

After three to four months of practicing Qi Gong, my cancer seemed to be under control and my liver function (ALP Test), improved. I now have more energy. My appetite is good and I can sleep well. I hope that by continuing to practice Qi Gong my cancer will be eliminated altogether. I believe Qi Gong helped me to minimize the side effects of chemotherapy by raising my white and red blood cells, and hemoglobin counts.

Cancer (Nose)

Jimmy
(Toronto, Canada)

Around 1964, I started doing Qi Gong in Hong Kong. Later, I was diagnosed with nose cancer and kept practicing during radiation. Practicing it, I always found it helped my health.

Fifteen years ago, after immigrating, I seriously began practicing Qi Gong again with Master Wu and learned how to send Qi to myself. It has made me feel empowered. I am cancer free and maintaining good health. I would just like to mention that Kidney Qi Gong is particularly very good for men.

Chest and Lung Problems

Chad Campbell
(Toronto, Canada)

For quite some time I have had recurring chest and lung problems, a bad cough and a lot of congestion seemed to follow me all the time. I had practiced Qi Gong for awhile myself, and then I decided to take formal classes, and after my first session, I felt my lungs and chest open and loosen, which after a week of sickness was a wonderful feeling.

After two more sessions, I felt healthy and vibrant. Being able to learn and practice the exercises makes me feel empowered. Being 18 years old it is a welcome change to be part of my own healing.

Chronic Fatigue Syndrome

V. Mac
(Toronto, Canada)

For 10 years, I suffered from Chronic Fatigue Syndrome. After one treatment and a lesson on relaxation with Qi Gong, I felt deeply relaxed more than I ever remembered feeling before. Also, when I continued to practice at home, the relaxed feeling happened each time I practiced. My sleeping also improved after the first treatment.

Chronic Pain due to Injury

Rose
(Toronto, Canada)

I found Master Teresa® through the internet, and it was after approximately three years of traditional physiotherapy I had done due to injuries sustained in a car accident. The traditional methods of physiotherapy only rehabilitated me so far and I still was not functional in everyday life. In addition to the injuries, I had Chronic Fatigue Syndrome, Fibromyalgia and chronic pain, so I started exploring the possibilities of Qi Gong. At the time it was still a bit too early to do my own practice so I had several one-on-one healing sessions with Master Teresa®, which was unbelievable. They are to date the only private healing sessions I've had where I wasn't wiped out all day and had to go home, unplug my phones and sleep. I was actually energized after Master Teresa's sessions and pain free for days and weeks after. Now I'm hoping to be able to start a private Qi Gong daily practice at home and hope to combat the chronic fatigue.

I hope this will encourage anybody with chronic fatigue or chronic pain due to injury or otherwise to seek out Qi Gong, because it really works.

Fibromyalgia

Vera Stern –Tai Chi and Qi Gong Instructor, Professional Harpist
(Toronto, Canada) www.verastern.com

Counting the years makes me aware of the ocean of time and the countless layers of painful emotions that were shed. In 1999, I was diagnosed with fibromyalgia. I was bedridden and had trouble sleeping due to having a lot of pain. My doctor prescribed Tai Chi. I did not know there was no cure.

I was a freelance musician and practiced everyday with the discipline of a musician, all movements filling up the need for renewed energy. I felt much better with the Tai Chi practice, enjoying it very much and I became a Tai Chi instructor. The pain and body improved a lot, but still I had a lot of pain.

My eye caught an ad of Master Teresa's Qi Gong in a health magazine. I pinned the ad on my fridge, but I didn't go to see her until a few years later.

I finally started Qi Gong with Master Teresa® in 2009 and began a new journey more miraculous than I ever imagined! My understanding of how the Qi flows completely changed. I enjoyed my Tai Chi movements with a new sense of the flow of energy and learned how to feel and collect Qi. My pain was reduced even more.

I realized that I can physically and mentally release my own pain with the new techniques I was learning with Master Teresa® Qi Gong. Emotionally, I also outgrew my accompanying state of constant worry, renouncing negativity and self-criticism. I started to have days without fibromyalgia pain and felt that life was possible without medication!

I took other Qi Gong classes with other famous masters to experience other styles of energy work. I truly feel the Qi Gong teachings and style I learned with Master Teresa® are simple and easy to learn. I formally joined her certification training, becoming a certified Instructor for Levels I and II. My practice paid off and after years of numbness, I felt my muscles come to life.

I have no more pain now! I am truly grateful for having the chance to learn this! And now am given the chance to share with my students.

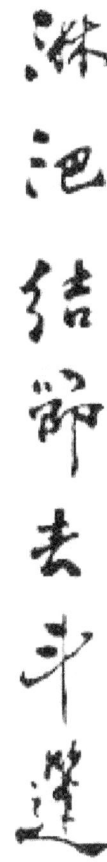

Clearing the lymphatic system eliminates cysts and fibroids and helps regain health.

Women's Issues

Cyst

Noah Sr. Chan
(Arizona, USA)

Growing up in a Chinese family, you were often surrounded by mythical tales of Kung Fu masters who possessed extraordinary fighting skills. And some masters had skills that transcended beyond the physical. The stories opened you up to a world of possibilities and the infinite potential that we all have inside of us. This narrative of unseen power was not exclusive to Chinese culture, but existed everywhere, for instance, "Trust in the Force" Luke Skywalker was told by his master in Star Wars.

I wanted to feel the force and have the force work for me and for the good of others. With each passing year, all children go through a stage of disillusionment. Cherished stories like Santa Clause are challenged and pried open to see it was nothing more than fantasy-driven narratives used to entertain our young and undeveloped minds. You see, as we become older and more wise the allegorical fantasies are replaced with hard science evidence, because that is the world of truth where you and I live, and so, we adapt to a paradigm of reality. We accept it without question. But inside, the intuitive voice screams the stories are true. Narratives of special healing abilities even pre-dates the time of Christ. In art, paintings and even stories written in stone tablets tells an ancestral history of gifted ones with abilities handed down from the heavens to heal and to comfort. Were all these stories a coincidence? A healthy mind is a skeptical mind as I am often reminded.

Even with the many stories of the miraculous that defy logic- in the end it was just that, great stories without evidence. Until I could see it for myself, I remained skeptical, drowning out the intuitive voice that told me otherwise. It was not until my wife was pregnant with our son Noah did all my existing ideas of reality get flipped completely on its head. Finding out you're having a baby can only be described as simply miraculous: the joy, excitement and of course, fear that accompanies first time parents is all too evident. Unfortunately, for us the joy and excitement were quickly extinguished by fear when our OB told my wife that she had a grapefruit-size cyst. It was in danger of bursting and could be life threatening to Noah. Surgery was out of the question -- it was extremely high risk. What were our options? My son's life was at risk. My critical mind was without an answer. Then the intuitive voice inside grew louder - the stories! What other option did we have?

Master Teresa® is a gifted and loyal student of a legendary Chinese Kung Fu Grandmaster and healer - the sole heir to Wu's Qi Gong lineage. It was time for me to see if the stories were finally true. Master Teresa's demeanor was of poise and great sensitivity, and matter of fact. She told my wife it was not an issue at all and not to worry; everything would be just fine. There was something different when she uttered those words. Throughout life we often hear empty words, people saying things without sincerity or depth. It was not the case with Master Teresa®. I felt an incredible ease, a truth and ultimately a faith in what she said was right. Noah was going to be just fine.

In a few short months, after my wife attended weekly private healing sessions, coupled with her own Qi Gong practice, the cyst was entirely gone. The doctor's only explanation was it happened by itself. But Noah, my wife and I know the truth - it was the stories.

The stories of great masters that are among us, that heals and comforts. Thank you, Sifu Teresa.

Cheryl Koenighauer
(Florida, USA)

This simple, powerful practice has had for me life-changing results.   After the first class, I could feel improvement in my neck that lasted for days. Each week forward, brought more noticeable physical improvement combined with a growing sense of self-love and appreciation. With each continued 6-week course, I''m feeling more empowered and using the methods to enhance my mind, body, spiritual connection.

I enjoy the experience of practicing and healing with Master Teresa and the supportive environment she has created within the classes. I'm inspired and grateful for women I've met in the classes as we share in each other's healing journeys. Love and Gratitude.

Hannah
(Toronto, Canada)

   I started Master Teresa's course for women. About 3 weeks later my naturopath told me that I don't need to take progesterone, estrogen and testosterone. I have stopped taking it for 6 weeks now and have no hot flashes or symptoms. The only thing I have done differently is Master Teresa's course. I will share with you that I was very very tired during the courses and participated only minimally and still got this great effect. I highly recomment Master Teresa and her courses.

Mary Shoemaker
(Michigan, USA)

   When I first signed up the women's qi gong. I had been suffering with a frozen shoulder for nearly a year and was scheduled for surgery. After a month of practicing a technique I learned in the class, my shoulder improved so much that I cancelled the surgery. I was amazed at how good I felt after each class and how much better I felt overall as I continued to practice. The diverse group of women striving to improve their health and quality of life kept me motivated. Master Teresa is an inspiration and a wonderful teacher and healer. I would recommend Women's Issues Qi Gong to women of all ages and cultures.

Maylynn Quan – Photographer
(Toronto, Canada) Www.Maylynnquan.com

   Master Teresa's Women's Qi Gong classes were exactly what I needed as I moved through so many challenges this past year; both physically and emotionally. It is rare and such a blessing to be mentored and lead by a female Qi Gong Master as this role was traditionally held by men alone. Having Master Teresa focus on our needs, as women, was a wonderful opportunity to learn, listen and nurture ourselves in a world where many of us are juggling multiple roles as caregivers and breadwinners. It was truly a gift to myself to be led by Master Teresa and to be a part of this wonderful group of strong women.

Depression

Anonymous
(Orlando, Florida)

My daughter was in high-school and a very good student. Suddenly her marks started dropping a lot, and then she began skipping school, and not talking to the family. She was very depressed. I met Master Teresa® at her workshop in Orlando. My daughter received an energy healing from Master Teresa® and immediately got a lot better. The next day she was willing to talk to the family, and the good news is her behavior improved ever since. She went on to college in the fall for about one month. Thank you so much!

Detoxification and Energy

Jaz
(Toronto, Canada)

I'm a nurse and I've always been interested in the alternatives and I found Qi Gong to be exceptionally helpful in sending energy to the body. For me personally, I have found that Qi Gong energizes me. It's a great detoxifier. My bowel movements improved tremendously, which means I'm detoxifying regularly. Since my energy level improved, I've achieved a lot more in my life being 50 with three kids and a very busy lifestyle. Qi Gong has been a lifesaver for me. I find that my lower back and knees have all improved thanks to Qi Gong. Thanks to Master Wu and Master Teresa® for bringing this to Canada.

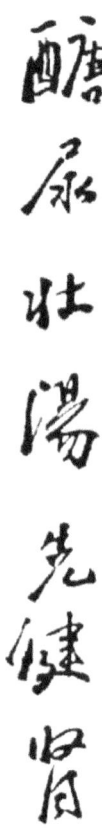

Boosting the kidney strengthens the libido affected by diabetes.

Diabetes

Brady Forsythe
(Burlington, Canada)

I have been off the diabetes medications now for over a month. This is the first time in 13 years. My weight dropped from 205 pounds since the first class to 190 pounds. Since taking Qi Gong, I have made it a mission to practice when I can, eat more natural foods and increase activity more. All these combined have made that much difference.

Energy Blockages (Physical and Emotional Issues)

Dunja
(Toronto, Canada)

I first met Master Teresa® at a Yoga show. Master Teresa® gave me 15-minute check-up, with which she sensed all my pain and blockages in exactly the correct places. I was amazed at her medical knowledge and intuition, and found her application of the Qi energy to diagnose my condition to such an accurate degree very intriguing. Even though she never had laid an eye on me or knew any of my medical history, she was able to correctly locate my blockages and point out some deep seated physical as well as emotional issues.

At this time in my life I was desperately seeking some healthy form of healing, which led me to Master Teresa's office for a private consultation. Master Teresa® guided me into a state of deep relaxation and through a series of visualization techniques, while at the same time performed her Qi treatment on me. I did not know what to expect, but cannot explain the immediate shift in my body and the great relief I felt when I left her office. After just a few treatments I felt such an improvement that I was convinced that I could only benefit from taking the workshops in order to learn how to apply some of the Qi Gong forms on my own.

I must say that using this ancient form of movements has been beneficial to my health and wellbeing on many different levels. Practicing the movements not only had a very calming and relaxing effect on my mind and body , but also resulted in better concentration, more clarity in my mind and a general feeling of balance and harmony. In short it just felt like a much better place to be in than before I practiced Qi Gong.

I've found Master Teresa's approach and techniques helped me to successfully exchange my bad habits for better behaviors conducive to supporting my career, family and overall lifestyle. Master Teresa® is truly a unique teacher in that her deep Qi Gong experience serves as a foundation for her continuous thirst for knowledge yet these attributes are complimented by a genuine empathy for her students and patients.

HEALING HORSE WITH COLIC

Julie Tirakian
(Michigan, USA)

The horse I am leasing was colicing severely. Colic is an EXTREMELY PAINFUL condition in horses' intestines that occurs suddenly and can be life threatening. The vet examination revealed a bowel impaction that was extremely hard to the touch. He (the vet) thought that surgery might be required and recommended that we not wait to take the horse to the university equine hospital 2 hours away.

I contacted Master Teresa and asked for her help. When we arrived at the university, the attending veterinarian found that the impaction was no longer hard and had softened a great deal. This meant that surgery might not be required and that the impaction could be cleared by oral administration of fluids, (the least invasive option). Attendants were also surprised that Bambi appeared to be so comfortable, given her condition. Master Teresa continued to send energy overnight. The next day we received word that Bambi was improving faster than expected, and that she would be released a day early. Since so much less intervention was needed, the hospital bill was LESS than HALF of the original estimate!

Amazing!! We are so grateful!

11. WU'S EYE QI GONG® HEALINGS

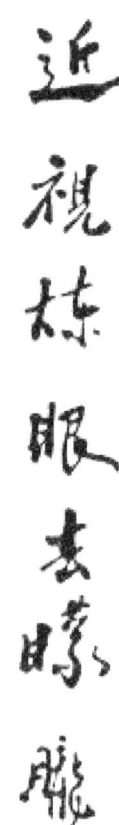

Wu's Eye Qi Gong® trains the eyes, clearing blurriness and myopia.

Use Your Eyes or Lose Them!
Wu's Eye Qi Gong®

C. Norman Shealy - MD, Ph.D.
President of Shealy-Sorin Wellness and Holos Energy Medicine Education
https://normshealy.com/

   The Eye Qi Gong has reduced my reading glass magnification.
I was introduced recently to Eye Qi Gong, and after the first class with Master Teresa, I suddenly realized that I do physical exercise of virtually every muscle in my body except those that move my eyes!

   Ordinarily our eyes are used at about 10% of their range of movement! Is this couch potato use of the eyes responsible for decreased visual acuity, cataracts and even macular degeneration? Certainly all other of the 5 basic senses are physically stimulated through a wide range of possibilities. Just as you need physical exercise at least 30 minutes 5 days a week; it seems logical and perhaps essential to do eye exercises 5 days a week!

   Intuitively and physically, after exposure to Eye Qi Gong, I urge you to consider it an essential health habit!

Childhood Blindness

Garry Tibbo - Nutritionist
(Toronto, Canada)

   My youngest daughter - my wife and I didn't know - when she was a little girl had no vision in one of her eyes. She was basically blind; however, the other eye had 20/20 vision. When she started school at approximately five years old, she had to have an eye exam. The doctor sent her to a specialist and the specialist said that she was guessing at the cue cards and basically, she had no vision. I had already been studying Qi Gong with Master Teresa® and she gave us a program in which to study and practice for my daughter, wife and I every morning before she went to school, or do what she had to do. After about one month, we went back to the same doctor and she had 20 percent vision in that one eye. Since then, we haven't practiced religiously or all the time, but my daughter at 13 years old reads books constantly and doesn't get headaches, or tired. Basically, there's no change in the eye, but it also has not gotten worse. She has vision in that eye, when before she had none. This is just one of the stories I could talk about.

My daughter's vision improvement is living proof. My older daughter had a stroke in her face with Bell's palsy and every time she opened her mouth to smile, her eye closed. Now she has no symptoms for almost 20 years. This is living proof. Qi Gong is something you should investigate.

Detached Retina

Dr. Roxanne Daleo, PHD – Health Psychology
(Harvard, Massachusetts) http://www.drroxannedaleo.com

I have a background in mind and body medicine, and realized that if I found the right teacher, I could use energy to assist in the healing of my eye. I had an unexpected medical emergency of a detached retina, and had to have surgery urgently to reattach it.

Natural healing is very important to me. I was introduced by my friend, Ed Dolezal, to Master Teresa® before, and felt I would like to experience her work. Therefore, I started to practice with her through a few telephone sessions. She taught me how to take my power back by practicing Qi Gong and healed with her Qi.

While feeling improved with the Qi Gong sessions, I was pressured to go for more surgery, which I did. My surgery was successful and the doctor was very impressed by my advanced healing. The attachment was almost perfect, solving over 80 percent of the problem. Altogether I had three eye surgeries, but I never stopped my Qi Gong practice.

Now I have recovered 85 percent of my vision, which is a miracle. Every time I visited the doctor, she was impressed with the speed of my eye recovery. Practicing Qi Gong regularly is indeed very good for my natural healing. Master Teresa® has a positive influence with my eyes!

I want to express my deep respect and appreciation to Master Teresa® for her assistance during my medical/surgical crisis. Thank you again, Master Teresa®, for your excellent care and gentleness in the way you were working with me to help me understand and trust more the power of our inner energies and the method of Qi Gong.

Dr. Roxanne Daleo (Dr.Roxie) has over 20 years experience helping children help themselves with stress-related disorders. A Health Educator who taught at Harvard University Health Services, she has successfully developed programs to foster your child's resilience, self-esteem and coping for a lifetime of wellness, wholeness and wisdom.

Glaucoma

Carlo Di Giovanni - Labour Relations Lawyer
(Toronto, Canada)

I suffered some vision loss from glaucoma and intraocular pressure. Since my diagnosis, I've been focused on doing everything I can to keep my eye pressure down. I take medicated drops, but I am also making changes to my lifestyle, including trying alternative healing approaches. I was referred to Master Teresa® Wu's Eye Qi Gong®Form and thought I would give it a try, not knowing what to expect. Right away I felt her energy and the comfort that came from her encouragement. She helped me to focus on a number, which was lower than any eye pressure reading I had after months of using my eye drop medication. Amazingly, at my next doctor's appointment, my eye pressure reading was exactly the number that Master Teresa® had helped me envision. I was very encouraged and will continue to supplement my medicine with Qi Gong practice.

Macular Degeneration

Dr. Nelson, MD
(Florida, USA)

A patient of mine had been experiencing severe eye pain as a result of macular degeneration. This pain prevented her from reading, that being one of her favorite activities. I taught this patient some very simple breathing, movement and visualization techniques that I had learned from Master Teresa®. After just a few weeks of practicing these exercises for only 15 minutes daily, this patient states that her eye pain is 90 percent improved and she can now read for several hours each day.

Keratoconus

Vince Larenza
(Ontario, Canada)

I have an eye condition, which involves the eye's shape to distort. This disease is called Keratoconus – a peaking form of the eyes that causes the distortion of sight. This condition cannot be corrected with glasses and there is no known cure. The only solution to see better is to wear contacts specifically designed for this condition, which can be quite uncomfortable, expensive, and in many cases, people never get used to wearing them. These contacts still do not promise to give excellent vision. The disease continues to progress, and in some cases, vision cannot be corrected anymore. The last resort would be eye transplants, which is the only real solution. However, donors are not easy to find and there is still no guarantee. I was wearing the contacts for a long time – at least four-to-five months with no change to my vision.

I began doing Qi Gong exercises and healing sessions. After a little more than a month, there were some changes. My vision changed and I have only gone through one pair of contacts since. My vision is still in flux, but there has been some improvement to 25-20 vision. The doctor has also found another way to improve my vision.

There are not enough words to describe how much I appreciate the healing power of Qi Gong.

Fear after a Trauma

Renate
(Toronto, Canada)

It is a FANTASTIC feeling to be safe and in tune with the horse again. I have missed that feeling for several years. Horseback riding has always been my sanity, my retreat. To feel one with the horse is an AWESOME experience and feeling. Thank you so much for getting me back on to that road. I still have work to do, but I am feeling the peace already. Thank you!

Traditional Chinese Medicine

Jireh Leung
(Toronto, Canada)

Being a Chinese born Canadian, learning about "Qi" is a difficult task and most certainly a hard concept to grasp. After exposure to its theories, and becoming a student in Traditional Chinese Medicine, I can say confidently now that it can turn complex ways of living, into simple ones. Wellness and longevity for example, is something that most want in their own lifestyle, but hard to maintain. I believe that having the understanding of Qi - recognizing the body as a vessel of energy, and always influenced by its environment - is crucial to healthy living.

Traditional Chinese Medicine can provide many answers to disease prevention and to longevity, and not surprisingly, Qi is at the heart of its practice. We first need to recognize that our minds, our bodies and our organs are very delicate. If an individual does not make the conscious choice to nurture their body and organs (the "Zang Fu 臟腑 or 脏腑"), he or she will suffer. We can also become less aware of the habits that prevent our bodies from healing effectively, if we do not make conscious choices that bring us to maintain a healthier life. This is unfortunate, but very commonly seen in cases where an individual suffers from chronic diseases.

My own first experience with Qi Gong came about two-and-a-half years ago, when I first practiced "Wu's Eye Qi Gong®", led by Master Teresa. I was honestly confused at that time. There was doubt in my mind and practices that conflicted with my understanding of 'health'. Needless to say, I dug a lot deeper, and realized that the Eastern approach to medicine was much richer in culture, than I ever imagined. Now, I practice Eye Qi Gong frequently after being refined by a great personal teacher. I have made adjustments in certain areas of my life, starting first with changing unhealthy eating, sleeping and working habits. These things eventually add to our own knowledge-bank and we have a responsibility to live it out, and educate the next generations to come.

Femur Fracture

Sarah Wells - Olympian
(Toronto, Canada)

I was injured for almost nine months and was at a point where I didn't know what else to do or how to heal myself. Being a national team athlete, I just wanted to get back on to the track. I was introduced to Qi Gong by a teammate and started working with Master Teresa® who helped heal my femur in my leg - a stressed fracture. After a month of working with her, I was back on to the track and working towards my goal of making the Olympics.

Every time I finished a session of Qi Gong, I would feel my body get a bit stronger than the way it was before I entered the room or started my session of Qi Gong. I believe that truly helped my success.

Also working with Master Teresa®; she taught me a strong lesson on how to connect my mind with my body and work with that energy to become in unison. I was able to use that lesson in my training and in my competitions. I encourage anyone who has not used Qi Gong to give it a chance, even though it isn't widely used.

Focus and Stress Reduction

Jason Leung - Head of Audience Marketing for Global Software Company

I started Qi Gong when I was studying in university over 10 years ago. My primary focus was career development and my initial motivation for Qi Gong was to relieve stress, have greater focus and relaxation. Currently, I am enrolled at Cornell-Queen's Executive MBA. What I came to realize is that beyond the superficial benefits that Qi Gong provide Master Teresa's coaching techniques helped me most significantly to make positive behavioral changes. Namely, I've found the plethora of self-help books; seminars and one-on-one coaching sessions tend to fall short at the stage when lasting change in habits is required. In contrast, I've found Master Teresa's approach and techniques helped me to successfully exchange my bad habits for better behaviors conducive to supporting my career, family and overall lifestyle.

Master Teresa® is truly a unique teacher in that her deep Qi Gong experience serves as a foundation for her continuous thirst for knowledge, yet these attributes are complimented by a genuine empathy for her students and patients. The term "open-minded" is used frivolously and generously in today's society, but I must confess that I have never understood its meaning in practice. Master Teresa® effortlessly exudes this quality, which allows her to understand and accept a student without judgment or presumption. The open dialogue and interaction that ensues, allows a student (if they are willing) to forgo the typical time-consuming, exhausting presence that occurs at the beginning and throughout a learning and healing journey. She dives right into the "good stuff".

Frozen Shoulders

Wing Fong - Computer System Programmer

I have been working in the Information Technology for over 30 years. I learned Qi Gong from Master Wu 16 years ago. It is a wonderful feeling when I practice it. Fifteen years ago, I developed frozen shoulders. Both my arms could not fully extend to both sides of my body and I could not raise them above my head. Master Wu worked on my shoulders three times; each time within the first couple of minutes, my shoulders were back to normal. So far, I have no pain – amazing! I am sure Qi Gong is good to everyone.

I am working on becoming a Qi Gong Instructor after my retirement, sharing the knowledge of Qi Gong in the communities.

Head Pain

Martin Tietz
(Czech Republic) http://www.martintietz.com

I work as an Engineer for TV studios worldwide. I have been interested in the martial arts and Eastern philosophies since I was young. I practiced Wushu for a short time at University. Then, I focused more on inner techniques such as Tai Chi and Yoga, and later on some forms of Qi Gong. I learned Qi Gong last year, and I have been practicing it regularly for longer than half of the year. I see this as a very easy, powerful and helpful technique for improving health. It helped me to reduce a head pain and better my eyesight. Regular practice has a remarkable benefit for personal and spiritual growth.

I recommend practicing Qi Gong twice a day for a few months. You will see significant benefits in your life. It is necessary to practice regularly! This exercise will bring you a lot of vital energy and a peaceful mind. I would like to thank to Master Teresa® for all the excellent work and efforts she has done.

Headache (Severe)

Aline Lohmann Chikude
(Brazil)

My main problem was a very severe headache, located in a very tiny spot at the right side of my head. The pain was getting stronger and stronger. A lot of tests were done, and finally the physician told me that there was nothing, and I should just try to find myself a hobby, and of course, take painkillers if I needed to. I was shocked and I told him that maybe there was a mistake. Something must be wrong since the pain was unbearable and every pain must have a root cause after all, right? The answer was once again "no, you have nothing".

About 12 years ago, I met Master Wu. I made an appointment for a healing session with him so he could diagnose this pain. I remember this day very well. I lay down and Master Wu took my hand and placed it on the area of my head and asked me if I was feeling the lumps. Yes, I did and there were many lumps! I didn't notice them before. My husband Kendi also felt them. Then Master Wu started the healing session. After he finished the session and I placed my hand on the area again, the lumps were gone! And so was my headache… unbelievable! I never felt that killing pain again. It was caused by stagnated Qi.

Of course the benefits of Qi Gong do not end there. I began practicing Qi Gong to help me relieve stress, sadness, pain, and on the other hand, to feel more alive, happy and content and full of energy. It helped me develop my perception and inner wisdom so that I could feel events before they happened. For example, avoiding a car accident (you can feel what the other driver intends to do, so you can be prepared to avoid the accident, or sense if someone is going to cross the street, so you can slow down and be prepared to hit the brakes). You can also help others or the environment by emitting, moving and circulating Qi. These are a few examples of what Qi Gong can do for us. I am very thankful to Qi Gong!

Migraines

Grade 10 Student

I remember having migraines and headaches since I was two years old. As I grew older, I was having them constantly. In the last two years, there was a particular kind of headache I had all the time and it never stopped. I stopped going to school, because the headaches became unbearable. Six weeks ago, my mother found Master Teresa®. She started to balance and teach me Qi Gong to practice at home. Every time I saw her, my headaches were less intense. My headaches are now 50 percent less and much easier to cope with. I find the practice of Qi Gong very useful and relaxing. The challenge is making ourselves start doing it. Once I start, I enjoy the practice. I plan to return to school soon!

Improved Concentration and Relaxation

Louis Hui

I am glad to have taken the step to learn Qi Gong with Master Teresa®. I was looking for a form of meditation that allowed me to increase my concentration, to relax, and to better manage the stresses of work and daily life. At first, I was skeptical of the principles of Qi Gong, given my education in science. But if anything, I accepted its principle if only for the ability to improve my concentration and relaxation. As I accepted the practice of Qi Gong, I am becoming aware of the other benefits it can provide for healthy mind and heart. I am only beginning my learning and practice now, but I look forward to continue developing my skills in Qi Gong and to improve the quality of my life.

Internal Bleeding

Nelly
(Toronto, Canada)

I found that the essence of Qi Gong is about responding instead of reacting to life-changing experiences. It helps to shift our consciousness in such a way that our decision-making shifts as well, and through that, we are generating Qi as well. So it's not always about eating healthy, although that's a huge part of it, but it's a combination of the mind, and how we choose to feel. Every feeling has a vibration, so after a couple of near death experiences, I had a choice to make at a soul level. That was when I shifted to soul consciousness and generating Qi to stay at a higher level physically. It allows the body to contain a greater amount of energy so you have time to make a shift in your life. So in that way it was life-changing for me.

I had 22 blood transfusions in about five months. The blood is also Qi. The Qi travels throughout the body through the blood, so I was losing so much blood that I had to be creative in not allowing that to happen anymore. There were a lot of insights that came with Master Teresa® giving extra Qi sessions to me. The medical doctors didn't know what to do with me. I was a very mysterious case. I was back and forth in emergency so many times. They even referred me to end-of-life care. But my bleeding completely stopped, which is a miracle. I practice Qi Gong every day.

Kidney (Failure)

My 88 year old father suffered from kidney failure and complained of low energy and lack of appetite. His balance was poor and he had difficulty walking. When he first met with Master Teresa® he could barely make it into her treatment room. After a healing session, he walked out of the room with a spring in his step! His breathing and energy levels has greatly improved.

Master Teresa® instructed him in ways to continue and improve his overall wellbeing. Her help is definitely improving his quality of life.

Kidneys (Weak)

Nancy

Since as long as I can remember, my kidneys have been weak. I would get up one to three times in a night to pee. After 10-to-12 hours of sleep, I was still tired and felt like staying in bed. I experienced dizzy spells and felt pressure in my head. Very often my brain would disconnect for short periods of one to three seconds.

Then I had the opportunity to attend Wu's Health and Fitness Qi Gong. I started practicing Qi Gong an hour a day. After three weeks, my brain stopped disconnecting and I have never again experienced the feeling of pressure in my head. I still sometimes get up to urinate, but not every night. Since practicing Qi Gong, I have more energy and happiness.

Lung Infection

David Bryan
(Toronto, Canada)

When I first met Master Teresa®, I had a lung infection caused by typical tuberculosis, which had persisted for two years. Long-term antibiotics prescribed by a Western respirology specialist had not succeeded in eliminating the infection. I felt discouraged, and was desperate to find some kind of treatment that would help me. Although I had no knowledge of traditional Chinese medicine, Master Teresa's calm and kindly manner inspired me to try receiving medical Qi Gong sessions from her, and I am very glad that I did.

Over a six week period of receiving medical Qi Gong sessions from Master Teresa®, and doing the internal Qi Gong exercises she recommended, my level of energy and sense of well-being improved greatly. I gained more from six weeks of Qi Gong than I had from over a year of the long-term antibiotic pharmaceuticals. I now practice Qi Gong exercises daily, and continue to learn more about how to use Qi Gong to improve health. I greatly appreciate the assistance that Master Teresa® has given me in moving into better health and vitality.

Panic Attacks

Ilana
(Israel)

A few months back, for the first time in my life, I started getting panic attacks. They began after a scary moment of choking after a meal and felt I could not breathe. I thought the experience had come and gone when suddenly a sensation of panic came over me. My throat tightened up, I had rapid heartbeat and numbness as I was driving home a few days later. I started to get scared and felt unsafe with every passing minute, not knowing when I would be able to breathe properly and being left alone in case I couldn't control it. I was constantly on the verge of tears and could not function. For the first time in my life I was truly terrified. My mother suggested Master Teresa® and I thought there was nothing to lose so I agreed. After the first session, as she told me to put my hand on my heart and explained how to calm myself, the notion returned in my mind that I was still in control.

After the second session, I started believing again that I could handle the situation and that there was nothing to be afraid of. By the third session I was smiling and so much more relaxed and she could sense it.

Since the first session, I didn't have an extreme attack, and whenever the feeling started to return, I immediately did as Master Teresa® advised: calm myself and wait patiently for my heart to go back to its normal pace. It took a few weeks until I wasn't thinking about it constantly, but even during those few weeks I wasn't scared to be alone. Words cannot describe how thankful I am at the quick recovery and simple methods that I could use at any given time, and not have to be dependent on anyone. I am once again relaxed and couldn't be happier.

Stage Performance

Robert Coxon Haig
(Quebec, Canada)

I've studied Qi Gong for five or six years and I perform music throughout the world, for audiences of 2,000 to 3,000 people. But I find that it really helps me just before I step onto the stage to do maybe five minutes of Qi Gong. I play so much better and I'm focused. All the notes are right and my hands play much faster, and the energy pours through me to the audience when I'm playing. It helps get the music out to the audience. It's quite beautiful, actually.

Shelli - Speaker
(Toronto, Canada)

I wanted to thank Master Teresa for helping me rearrange my energy. I was a mess when I walked in her door and felt super calm when I walked out. I have come to realize that I need to do a lot of work surrounding self love. My last talk on the stage was amazing. It was 10 times better than my highest hope.

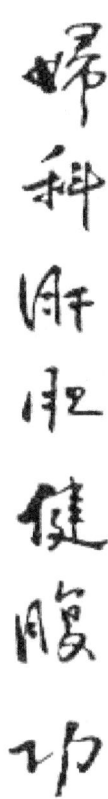

Abdominal Qi Gong improves gynecological health, liver and gall bladder.

Infertility

Carol
(Mississauga, Canada)

I wished that I knew Qi Gong 8-10 years ago. My husband and I had problems conceiving a baby and we were once very disappointed. We went through many infertility procedures before conceiving a baby. Going through all the medical treatments felt like an emotional rollercoaster!

With my experiences with Qi Gong now, I really think that a husband and wife getting involved in Qi Gong will really calm down the couple's energy while going through all the medical procedures. I definitely believe that if couples do Qi Gong together it increases the chances of conception. If we knew of Qi Gong, we would have coped with the emotional turmoil better. We would have gone through the process a lot better.

My husband commented that all the medical procedures we went through to conceive a baby didn't consider our emotions, just the physical body. He said that he felt so emotionally stressed seeing me suffer emotionally and physically. I remember feeling bad when I found out that I could not donate blood, because my blood was not good from taking all the drugs.

For me, I feel that Qi Gong really balances and helps me to see things differently. I'm more in tune with people, customers, my husband and family. I feel that I have a calming effect on those around me, which is an unexpected good result. My husband also notices that I am more balanced emotionally, dealing with things better, becoming a better person, which is helping our relationship.

However, some people are not very open to change or energy. Some get it and some do not. For example, my boss seems to like me when I am angry rather than normal. Others do not understand my change and cannot figure out why I am behaving so calm. I feel that they are afraid of my growth.

Pak Ho
(Mississauga, Canada)

I had my first and only son when I was 60 years old. It was a miracle and truly a gift!

I started practicing Qi Gong, because I was getting up about four or five times at night to go to the bathroom. It was very tiring and I had no sex drive. The nightly urination condition gradually improved with the help of Qi Gong, especially the Kidney Qi Gong. My wife who is 20 years younger than me also practiced Qi Gong for her own health. About 5 years later, my wife got pregnant and gave birth to our son. I am most grateful to Qi Gong!

Menstrual Pain and Pelvic Inflammatory Disease (PID)

Rosie
(Toronto, Canada)

In early January 2013, I began seeing Master Teresa® for a medical condition that I was struggling with for almost two years.

In October 2011, and again in early March 2012, I was hospitalized with severe abdominal pain and a persistent high fever of 39 degrees. I was diagnosed with Pelvic Inflammatory Disease (PID) at the time of hospitalization. The first hospital stay lasted 4 days, but the second hospitalization lasted 10 days due to complications, because the infection progressed to my lungs. Both times the infection was treated with a cocktail of antibiotics.

I always had female issues of one sort or another. My periods were never regular, but when I did have them, there was significant discomfort. Since my hospitalization with PID, my periods have become extremely painful with persistent, almost-daily light spotting in between my periods. This made my daily life uncomfortable and quite unpleasant.

I had two in-person sessions with Master Teresa® and a few over-the-phone sessions. After my first session, the spotting ceased by the next morning. I was rather shocked that any progress could have happened so quickly. I have to admit that I was, at first, a bit skeptical, but I still remained hopeful. Throughout the weeks that followed, I did have some spotting, but it was not persistent and all the discomfort was gone. About two and a half weeks since my first session with Master Teresa® my period came. I was caught a bit off guard as there was no pain or cramping as usual.

In fact, my pelvic area felt unusually light. My entire period was so unlike any other period I had ever experienced. I did have some discomfort, but I didn't require any pain medication or bed rest. In fact, my daily routine was unaffected by what my body was going through - this was a first! I am so grateful for Master Teresa® and her gift. This is life changing for me.

Post-menstrual Symptom (PMS)

Brenda
(Toronto, Canada)

Energy fascinates me, especially its paradoxical nature of remaining constant yet being in a perpetual flow of change from one form to another. A few examples of these ever present yet endless energy transformations are; the food chain, the life cycle, seasonal weather systems and human mythologies. One of my favorite mythologies is the transformation of a person after a remarkable experience – that, according to the Encarta Dictionary – is interpreted as a sign that a necessary change is needed in the way that a person lives their life. Think about Dickens's legendary Ebenezer Scrooge in *A Christmas Carol* or the infamous Grinch in *The Grinch Who Stole Christmas* by Dr. Seuss and you've got the idea. These powerful metaphors of change are a reminder that anyone can better their life if they are willing to do the energy work. I like the idea that a person can indeed encourage a positive change in their hearts and lives by eating wholesome food, staying active, remaining interested in life and practicing time-tested techniques like positive self-talk, Yoga, Tai Chi or Qi Gong. Applying these healthy habits can improve, balance, heal and elevate one's life force.

Several weeks before my initial meeting with Master Teresa, my lower abdomen and colon area felt blocked. It was an unusual feeling that I couldn't quite figure out. I wasn't constipated or experiencing PMS. I had already reached menopause two and a half years earlier. During the introductory session of Qi Gong with Master Teresa®, Master Teresa sent energy to the small assembly, while explaining how we store pleasant memories, thoughts and negative ones in our torsos. Immediately I felt a sharp, intense pain on my right side that caused me to wince. Noticing this, Master Teresa sent healing energy to me and the pain subsided. That night I still felt blocked, and when I woke up the next morning with post-menopausal bleeding, I knew something extraordinary had happened. Coincidence, possibly, or an early indicator of a health issue uncovered by the Qi Gong balancing session. I followed this health issue up with a few private Qi Gong sessions with Master Teresa, my GP, and an ovarian ultrasound. The pain left and all was well and is well.

That first experience, as well as the few private and group sessions that followed, were truly mind body energy opening for the better. As of today, I'm happy to say I continue to practice Qi Gong online with Master Teresa and a group of welcoming women.

Pinched Nerve

Philip Malkarous

I had a pinched nerve in my shoulder, which caused quite a bit of pain all the way down my arm to my fingers. The pain became worse and worse and it felt like my arm was on fire. I got anti-inflammatory pills from my doctor and went to a chiropractor, but the pain was getting very bad. A friend suggested that I see Master Wu. I took their advice and had two treatments with Master Wu the next day. I was in so much pain when Master Wu first touched me I thought I would jump off the table and run away. I tried to breathe through the pain, but about 10 minutes into the treatment I could not believe what was happening. My pain was almost all gone!

Master Wu asked me to sit up and I could not believe how good I felt. I came back for a second treatment later that day and felt even better. That night I was finally able to sleep. I continued with more treatments and I am amazed at how quickly the pain has gone.

Psoriasis

Annie

I used to have 80 percent of my body covered with psoriasis for many, many years. Now after seeing Master Teresa®, I am almost psoriasis free!

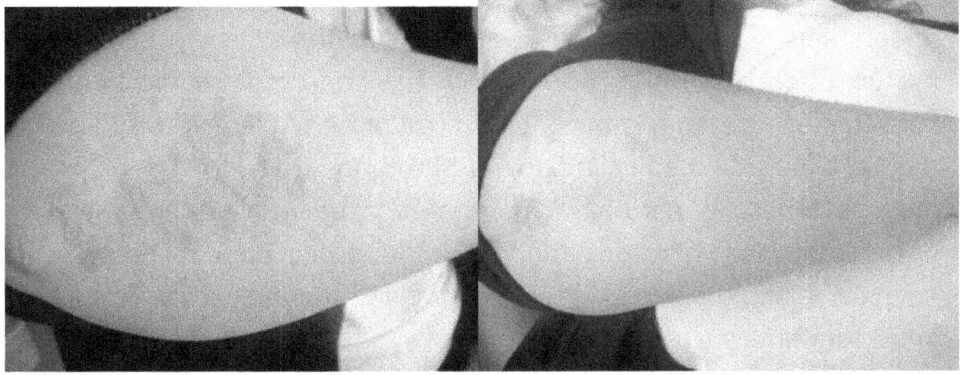

Before   After

Reduced Sciatica Pain

I was recommended by my naturopath to go and see Master Teresa®. Yes, like everybody else, I was desperate. The pain in my legs and my back made sleeping at night almost impossible for a full night's sleep. Desperation actually brought me here, but just after two treatments, I felt lighter. My pain was somewhat gone for at least a day. It came back the next day, but then I had another appointment, so I was optimistic, good actually and excited to go to the next appointment. Now I'm only on appointment four, but I can tell you that sciatica, which is so painful, down the legs and back is gone! It's just unbelievable! And now I'm looking forward to other ailments that are bothering me being treated by Master Teresa®. I actually have no doubt that she is going to fix them for me. Here I am, excited and anxious to have my next appointment. It's an amazing, amazing treatment! Amazing!

Relationship Harmonization

Erika and Andrew

We were in the middle of a tornado of patterns, and though we talked, etc., we couldn't seem to move beyond them and let go. The relationship harmonization was a blessing on so many levels. We healed individually and as a couple, which naturally restored harmony. The experience brought a deep understanding, allowing more awareness and tools to help transform and nurture our relationship(s). Though we have open communication and work hard to move through knots and patterns, it was Master Teresa's support and nature, alongside the healing power of Qi Gong that allowed the process to move effortlessly – naturally. Thank you for the blessings. We feel we have gotten more than harmonization out of our process and recommend it to all couples. Again, thank you for supporting and sharing with us at such an important time – true riches.

Severe Tendonitis

Margaret
(Aurora, Canada)

Our body is like a battery. Our blood is like the fluid in the battery. Qi is like the energy flow that charges the battery. When all three elements are in harmony, the body (the battery) functions properly.   We recharge our body energy through meditation and breathing exercise.

I started my journey with Qi Gong about 15 years ago. At the time my body was broken, my spirit low and naturally I had no Qi. My health was bad. Apart from constant headaches from a stressful life, broken home, money issues and also suffering from tendonitis, it took Master Wu almost four months to heal my crippling tendonitis. Soon enough, I started practicing Qi Gong. I wanted to make sure my tendonitis would not return and practicing it is what I can do to control my life.

It took a bit of time. Soon enough, I noticed that I mentally improved; my outlook in life got better. I am not as annoyed and bitter as before. Qi Gong must have harmonized my inner body.

Swelling In The Body

Dawn
(Toronto, Canada)

I did the QiEnergyPlus® weekend with Master Teresa®. It's been a life-transforming event. I was able to actually feel the Qi and the energy in the room. I feel transformed already and more open going forward. I've been able to sleep when I struggled to sleep. I fall asleep without realizing it.

Also, my legs weren't swollen. Usually in the mornings I'd wake up feeling dizzy and nauseous; I didn't feel any of that. Instead I'm energized and I actually feel encouraged and really happy that I did it.

Funnily enough, our bodies get conditioned so much that our body screams for help. Qi Gong does come to the rescue. Just meditate and think Qi and Qi will come to you.

Thyroid Disease

Lillian Gagic – Qi Gong Instructor
(Toronto, Canada)

I was working as a Project Manager in big corporation for over 13 years. As most of us do, I was neglecting my health and the messages my body was sending daily. I got to a point where my thyroid gland started growing a tumor and the left thyroid was removed in 2003. I was given synthetic hormones to "help" keep the right thyroid healthy. Those hormones didn't work as expected. The right thyroid started to grow a tumor as well. It was diagnosed in 2008, and that was the point when I decided to take responsibility for my health and life.

I was introduced to Master Teresa Yeung in January 2009. After completing Level I and Level II Qi Gong QiEnergyPlus® workshops, I immediately enrolled into the Instructor's training. Daily practice since February 2009 helped me improve my health. The tumor on the right thyroid and countless cysts in my entire body disappeared, stress slowly dissolved and everyday life improved. Seeing how beneficial the daily practice was for me, I decided to help others by teaching Qi Gong. In March 2010, I graduated from the General Qi Gong Instructor Level I and certified to represent the Institute to teach the Wu's Health and Fitness Qi Gong Form.

Today, I still use Qi Gong practice as a remedy for any pain, headache, discomfort or stress. Qi Gong helps build inner strength and, with that, everyday life becomes enjoyable and fulfilled with peace and happiness.

Ulcerative Colitis

Stephane Corre – Fa Qi Si
(Toronto, Canada)

I started Qi Gong early 2011 with Lillian Gagic, a Qi Gong instructor and one of Master Teresa® students. I learned Qi Gong Level I form and practiced it on and off for several months.

I met Master Teresa® at the 2012 Yoga Show in Toronto, which renewed my interest in learning and practicing Qi Gong. I then attended the QiEnergyPlus® Advanced Self-Healing Rebalancing four-hour workshop with Master Teresa® in mid April 2012 to help me rebalance.

In May 2012, I attended the Wu's Eye Qi Gong® Intensive workshop in order to improve my vision. I am now practicing Qi Gong twice a day, the Qi Gong for Men® form along with the Wu's Eye Qi Gong® after getting up in the morning and the Wu's Eye Qi Gong® at night before going to bed. Qi Gong helped me reconnect with my body and find a better inner peace and, therefore, allowed me to better manage my Ulcerative Colitis. It also helped me to be more in tune with my body and emotions, allowing me to approach day-to-day life challenges in a much more positive and relaxed way. I am really thankful for finding Qi Gong and also for all the help from Master Teresa® on my journey of improving myself through Qi Gong.

I graduated from Master Teresa's Fa Qi Si Program in November 2012, and I am now a Qi Energy Healer. This program taught me the tools and techniques to be able to heal myself and others, especially my family and significant other. I am currently in the process of promoting my own practice.

After my first weekend of the Fa Qi Si Program, I went for my usual acupuncture session and, for the first time none of the needles were poky. I also went to see my naturopath for my regular supplements check and my body no longer needed a couple of them, which I had been taking for years.

This year, I feel that my ulcerative colitis, that has been troubling me for 18 years, is in remission and finally healing! Practicing Qi Gong every day replaced my need for acupuncture sessions. When I saw my eye doctor in February

2012, he told me that my prescription was now too strong for my eyes. I haven't been wearing my glasses since then and do feel that my vision is improving!

At the 2012 Whole Life Expo and the 2013 Yoga Show, at Master Teresa's booth, I sent Qi and cleared people's pain and anxiety away without touching them!

Qi Gong changed my life in a really fulfilling way and has become a self-improvement journey for me.

Weakness In Right Arm

Grace Chan
(Toronto, Canada)

My brief experience with Qi Gong healing from Master Teresa® was encouraging. My right (dominant) arm felt really weak. I had to use both hands to pick up a hard-cover book. Sometimes it felt numb and cold, while my left hand was warm. After I went to Master Teresa® a few times, the strength gradually came back.

Weakness From Car Accident

Carol
(Mississauga, Canada)

I am professional woman, working as a Medical Sales Consultant for 18 years. I am very sensitive and naturally drawn to good energy. About three years ago, I visited an anti-aging show with my in-laws and was attracted to Master Teresa® Qi Gong booth. I was amazed by Master Teresa® body scan, telling me that I was weak in my body pertaining to a car accident I had about eight months ago. I felt that Qi Gong was the right thing for me to start doing and see how it might support my healing.

I started to get one-on-one sessions with Master Teresa® and felt my pain dissipate and lessen about 50-to-75 percent every time I had a session. Then I took Qi Gong classes and brought my loving husband along to the class, but he does not really feel like practicing, which is just fine with me. I have been faithfully practicing Qi Gong since and continued to have more one-on-one sessions with Master Teresa Yeung.

Wheelchair Healing

Q. Simmons
(Miami, Florida)

I am 45 years young and confined to a wheelchair due to a spinal cord injury that has made me paraplegic at level of T7 20 years ago. I found that Master Teresa's classes have provided me with immediate benefits and proof that this is a healing modality I will definitely pursue to practice further. The first day was intense because it required lots of upper body movement that I was not accustomed to. The following day, I was surprised that, after only three hours sleep the previous night (I was in the emergency room with my mom), I had plenty of energy to participate. Usually after a night spent awake, and sitting in my wheelchair, my feet and ankles would swell to resemble loaves of bread, but I had no swelling after Qi Gong. I acquired pain below my right shoulder blade near my spine – very near the site of my original injury. Master Teresa® worked on me, sending energy to this site. I have not had pain here in a very long time.

Master Teresa® said, "Qi Gong reminds the body of its original energy" and I believe my body did just that. The following day, the pain was gone. The pain is a memory. I wasn't sure what happened for those few hours.

13. SERVICES TO THE COMMUNITY

Arthur Lockhart - Executive Director - The Gatehouse
(Etobicoke, Canada) http://www.thegatehouse.org

I wholeheartedly support the work of Master Teresa®. Qi Gong is becoming an essential process we share with the participants at the Gatehouse. The process is powerful on so many levels: physical, mental and emotional. Qi Gong is a process that invites participants to uncover the tremendous healing strength that is within each and every one of us. I am grateful for the insightful teachings of Master Teresa®.

Gatehouse offers support groups and programs for child, youth, parents and adult survivors of childhood sexual abuse. It is a friendly neutral location for police officers and Children's Aid Workers to conduct interviews during child abuse investigations.

Many more community events / services have benefited from Master Teresa's Qi Gong, such as:

- Healing Conferences
- Hospitals
- Mental Health and Autism services
- Retirement homes / residences
- School Boards
- Street Mission
- Universities

14. QI GONG JOURNAL

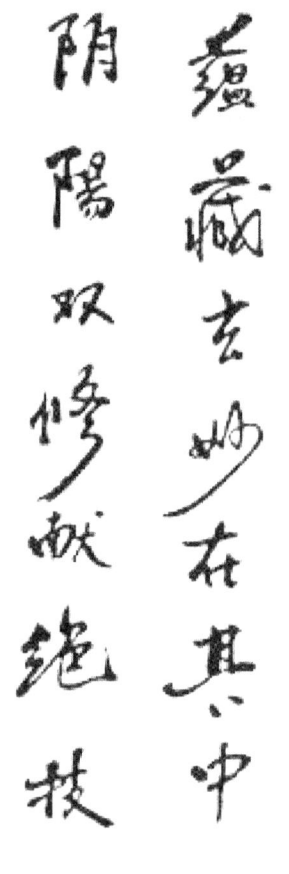

x

Yin (feminine) and Yang (masculine) are practiced together for best performance; great secret, mysterious wisdom exists within the Qi Gong practice.

If you maintain a Qi Gong practice once or twice a day, for 5-to-20 minutes for 100 days, it is a good start and you will be surprised by the great change! Take an experimental attitude and practice every day. You have nothing to lose.

Here are a few points to consider:

- It is important to do Qi Gong every day as the body needs Qi energy regularly to improve immunity.
- It is good to practice twice a day.
- It is usually fine to practice even when we are sick, for example, having a cold or fever.
- It is best to practice Qi Gong in-between meals.
- Start every day with a glass of water, then Qi Gong.
- Because Qi Gong is very energizing, it is not recommended to practice before going to bed, with the exception of "Wu's Eye Qi Gong® Form.
- Some students may yawn during practice, as they release negative Qi and tiredness.
- You may also feel tired during the practice as you clear negative energy out of your body.
- Please remember to drink 6 to 8 glasses of water a day, follow a healthy diet and get proper rest.
- If you have any health concerns about practicing Qi Gong, please consult your physician.
- Before starting your Qi Gong journey, complete the following pages to mark the milestones: the beginning, middle and end of the 100 days. Hopefully, you will continue beyond that, because the practice has transformed your life in a positive and uplifting way.
- BEFORE BEGINNING, get a notepad of some sort. There are many mobile apps to assist with note taking or creating lists of information. Otherwise, you can always go to a dollar store and pick something up there too!

FIRST 30 DAYS

Describe how you are currently feeling, both physically and emotionally. Physical: Write down any symptoms / medicines / pains. When do they occur?

Morning

Afternoon

Evening

Overall energy: Low / up and down / relatively well. Please describe:

Emotionally, how are you feeling?

What are your main thoughts?

Is there anything upsetting you? What is the cause of the stress / worry / anxiety?

Make a wish. Describe what will make you feel happier. For example, better health, a loving relationship or having your dream job.

Make a check mark after you have done your practice each day. For Example:

Morning Practice			Afternoon/ Evenings	
Example: ✔ 20 min			**X - not** this evening	
1	2	3	4	5
6	7	8	9	10
11	12	13	14	15
16	17	18	19	20
21	22	23	24	25
26	27	28	29	30
31				

SECOND MONTH

Describe how you are currently feeling, both physically and emotionally. Physical: Write down any symptoms / medicines / pains. When do they occur?

Morning

Afternoon

Evening

Overall energy: Low / up and down / relatively well. Please describe:

Emotionally, how are you feeling?

What are your main thoughts?

Is there anything upsetting you? What is the cause of the stress / worry / anxiety?

Make a wish. Describe what will make you feel happier. For example, better health, a loving relationship or having your dream job.

Make a check mark after you have done your practice each day. For Example:

Morning Practice			Afternoon/ Evenings	
Example: ✔ 20 min			**X - not** this evening	
1	2	3	4	5
6	7	8	9	10
11	12	13	14	15
16	17	18	19	20
21	22	23	24	25
26	27	28	29	30
31				

THIRD MONTH

Describe how you are currently feeling, both physically and emotionally. Physical: Write down any symptoms / medicines / pains. When do they occur?

Morning

Afternoon

Evening

Overall energy: Low / up and down / relatively well. Please describe:

Emotionally, how are you feeling?

What are your main thoughts?

Is there anything upsetting you? What is the cause of the stress / worry / anxiety?

Make a wish. Describe what will make you feel happier. For example, better health, a loving relationship or having your dream job.

Make a check mark after you have done your practice each day. For Example:

Morning Practice			Afternoon/ Evenings	
Example: ✔ 20 min			**X - not** this evening	
1	2	3	4	5
6	7	8	9	10
11	12	13	14	15
16	17	18	19	20
21	22	23	24	25
26	27	28	29	30
31				

FINAL 10 DAYS

Describe how you are currently feeling, both physically and emotionally. Physical: Write down any symptoms / medicines / pains. When do they occur?

Morning

Afternoon

Evening

Overall energy: Low / up and down / relatively well. Please describe:

Emotionally, how are you feeling?

What are your main thoughts?

Is there anything upsetting you? What is the cause of the stress / worry / anxiety?

Make a wish. Describe what will make you feel happier. For example, better health, a loving relationship or having your dream job.

Record Additional / Final Thoughts / Observances

15. FREQUENTLY ASKED QUESTIONS

Why is this book has so many testimonials and so little on how to practice Qi Gong?

For anything to change, we must first change ourselves.

This book is helping you to see the value of a simple Qi Gong practice of "Wu's Health & Fitness Qi Gong" that works. It has created miraculous healing to millions of people. The journey of our students will provide you the encouragement to see your own possibilities. You are and can learn to be in charge of your health physically and emotionally with our teachings. The movements we put down in this book is tremendously important to you. Please respect its simplicity and results will be obtained with persistance.

Join Master Teresa and her team teachings in her online school, YouTube and in other social media platforms.

She does teach online workshops live and offers free consultation.

Who Is Suitable To Practice Qi Gong?

Qi Gong can be practiced by anyone who is willing to learn and practice. If you have an illness, Qi Gong can help you to fight your disease and get well. If you have no sickness, Qi Gong can enhance the overall wellbeing of your body by strengthening your immune system.

Why Would I Learn Qi Gong From A Qi Gong Master?

People who have practiced energy work know the actual feeling of energy. Some feel warmth and tingling in their hands, while others feel something magnetic. These are common feelings, but this is not enough. Other people are pleased and very satisfied with this little Qi energy feeling, but what about those who want more?

We need the best to be instilled from a Master. Our Qi needs to be initiated by a Qi Gong Master or Qi Master before it can really work and achieve fast results. Where the mind is, the Qi will be there. When Qi arrives, healing will be enhanced. Qi Gong is the key to understand the "vast" or "big" knowledge of Qi. It requires time and much training to embrace the essence as to how the energy truly flows.

The Chinese will not casually learn Qi Gong from just any teacher. They understand and value a teacher's role while working with the Qi. They know practice is one thing, but focused practice with a master of Qi Gong will give better results. You will have more Qi if you learn from a teacher with more Qi. You will even have more Qi with a master who can project Qi. Master Teresa® learned directly from the source of Qi - China. Grandmaster Wu achieved the highest official Qi Gong title, the Chinese Talent Bank, and participated in the selection of Qi Gong Masters to join the Talent Bank during that tenure. His teachings and Qi are phenomenal. Master Teresa®, being his only successor, received the Master's Qi almost daily for over 10 years. Learning daily and watching him perform daily healings too. Master Teresa® now carries the torch, as she is heir to thousands of years of Qi Gong study and refinement. Her knowledge and Qi is one of a kind.

Why Is It Good To Learn From Master Teresa®?

Master Teresa® Qi Gong originally comes from China. Grandmaster Wu was a member of the Chinese Qi Gong Talent Bank. For the last thirty years, the Government of the Peoples' Republic of China has been conducting intense scientific studies and founded the Chinese Qi Gong Talent Bank for the Science Research Academy of Chinese Qi Gong and the Exchange Service Centre for the Science Research Academy of Chinese Qi Gong in Beijing (Peking). The research findings have demonstrated and proven the benefits of Qi Gong and its healing power. Master Teresa Yeung is the successor to the Wu's Qi Gong lineage. She has unique ability to see and scan energy. She has been sharing the teachings of Qi Gong for 24 years helping all kinds of healing throughout those years.

Grandmaster Wu said:

"Even if you go to China, you cannot learn any better."

Master Teresa's Qi energy carries a medicinal QiSignature™ that promotes healing. She possesses that fine-tuned Qi energy passed down from several masters. Master Teresa® teaches like no other. She wants us to learn how to self-maintain and self-heal. She delivers Qi demonstrations in all classes to show and embrace the power of the Qi in each student. Students who have experienced Master Teresa® will commonly comment that the energy she creates in the room is not only palpable but Qi energy they never experienced before. Why not join and feel her Qi traveling throughout the classroom or even over the phone?

What Do You Feel In A Qi Gong Class?

Learning Qi Gong is not about some movements or which forms. It matters who is your teacher. It matters if you are making that Qi, which promotes your self-healing and immunity. In our class, Master Teresa® connects with universal Qi, collects it and sends it to the students.

Simple to understand teaching method, correct posture and subtle positioning of movements, help you understand and feel how to move the Qi energy in your body quickly. Master Teresa has the ability to read the energy of the student's body, senses the blockages and guide students how to move forward better and faster.

She sends out Qi to balance the students' body physically and emotionally. It is common for students to feel calm and relaxed Qi energy in their hands and body, vibrational pulsing and magnetic feelings. Some tightness, aches and pains, even swelling are reduced.

I Have a Hard Time Sitting Down. How Can I Practice?

Some people have said that since they cannot sit still, they cannot focus, and thus, cannot do Qi Gong. Please understand that when you first practice Qi Gong, you may have trouble focusing and emptying your thoughts. The ongoing practice of Qi Gong gradually trains you to focus, empty your thoughts and develop patience. A good teacher can help you to enjoy your practice and you will love the experience of peacefulness.

16. MASTER TERESA'S CLASSES, PROGRAMS ONLINE & PERSONAL SESSIONS

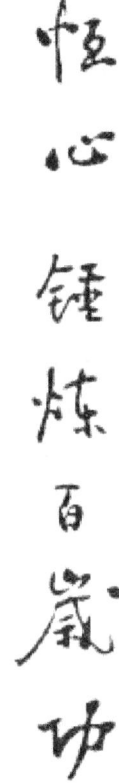

Practice Qi Gong with faith, dedication and perseverance to achieve its great reward: a happy, long and healthy life.

Master Teresa® classes and programs are easily accessible to students in-person, online, one-on-one sessions, in groups or remotely by phone, Skype and Zoom.

PURELAND QI GONG®

Master Wu once said to me, "The colour green comes from the blue colour". What he meant was blue represents the teacher and green represents the student. The student improves upon the information taught by the teacher.

After Master Wu's crossing into the spirit world, I explored what was missing in our practices, adapted and improved upon the teaching methods and designed new programs. The Ancient Chinese Fa Qi Healing is a new certification training that is based upon the teachings of the I-Ching, my insights and experiences in Chi healing.

Pureland Qi Gong® is a system of new easy-to-master Accelerated Chi Gong Techniques™ intention-based practice, which expedites the traditional method of making, collecting and cultivating the Qi energy and balancing emotions.

It contains the ancient secrets of masters living in the Chinese "sacred tall mountain", including Wu's Hunyuan Gong® and new science. It is like an old computer program, but enhanced to perform better and faster.

The techniques we use have more focus on training our intentions on how to move the energy to achieve the best results. She and her team are compassionate remote healers.

Here are some of popular Qi Gong:

- Wu's Eye Qi Gong®
- Wu's Health and Fitness Qi Gong™
- Heart Chi Gong to Balance Emotions
- Money Chi Gong to attract money

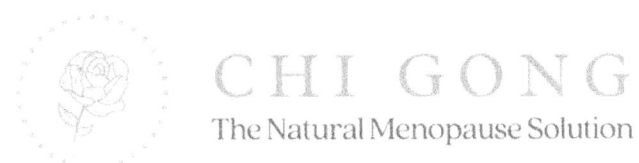

CHI GONG
The Natural Menopause Solution

The USA 2022 statistics showed that 1 and 8 women will be diagnosed with breast cancer and it is the No. 1 killer for women. Master Teresa Yeung's younger sister died of breast cancer and then expanded to brain cancer. She did not make it to 40 years old and left 2 young children. Before she was sick, she was given the opportunity to practice Qi Gong but she refused doing it. When she lost her vision to see clearly during chemo, she then started to practice and see again.

After 27 years of Chi Gong (Qi Gong), Master Teresa's insight are women must start practicing her Qi Gong for women's issues by menopause time to give enough time to heal the body.

She concludes that traditional Qi Gong is not good for grief nor really help to expedite the healing of menopausal symptoms. She said that because she was in tremendous grief when her master crossed and she also felt terrible during menopause. She only felt better each time after she organized the Qi Gong practice and created new ways of moving the Chi.

Most people would not realize that Qi Gong has been created by men masters as masters have always been men for thousands of years. The great teachers hid in the mountains. Students travelled to mountains to seek teachers. Women stayed home to be the caretaker, cooking, sewing and giving birth to more boys. To this date, Qi Gong masters are still usually men.

As a rare female master, Master Teresa, 65, she is now focusing on women to conquer the struggle during peri-menopause, post-menopause and beyond. Her offer is:

Put the Pain and Discomfort in the Past with Chi Gong
Digital 5-Module Course
Live 7-Week Classes, Recordings and Bonuses
12-Month Gold Membership

Chi Gong: The Natural Menopause Solution also has an **Affiliate Program**. She invites collaboration and professionals to help share her work. She loves to join your events as a speaker. Please check out:

www.ChangeTheEnergyKeepTheChange.com

REMOTE HEALING ON ZOOM

INSTRUCTORS PROGRAMS

Digital Course or In-Person

Master Teresa Yeung believes that many people can be trained to be "Qi energy practitioners". During Covid, she has trained over 34 practitioners to do Zoom Chi Balancing Sessions. Her programs go for 4 months to 6 months:

- Overall Chi Balancing
- Chakras Balancing
- 5 Element Chi Balancing
- Reduce Pain Balancing
- Improve Sleep Balancing

She teaches empaths not to take on other people's energies.

Her love has expanded to help animals. "Using Chi to Heal Pets" is vital teachings

.

Remote Qi Balancing Sessions

A private session is a good way to jumpstart your healing. As it is personal, the session will be given according to your needs. Master Teresa has a unique ability in which she scans your body for physical, emotional and energetic blockages. Even remotely, she actually sees and senses the negative energies and blockages. She has ability to guide you how to move forward in your life based on the energy messages of your body. She knows exactly where to go and is a great mentor for many people. The session is usually done remotely for emotional clearing and balancing.

She offers free online consultation:

purelandinternationalqigong.setmore.com/masterteresa

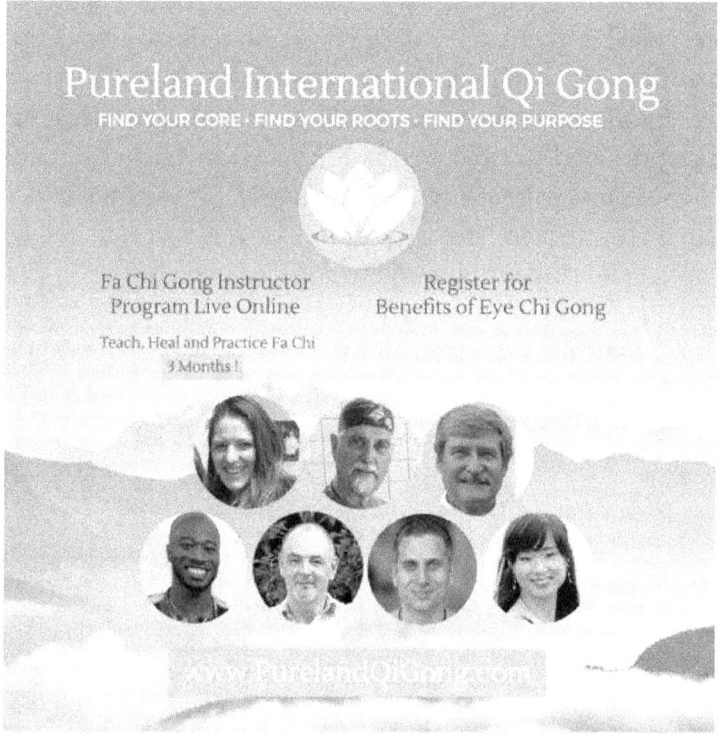

I did this beautiful online live online Fa Chi Gong Instructor course by Master Teresa Yeung, and I became a certified Qi Gong instructor. Amazing that it can be done online! But it really works. I highly recommend this course if you want to learn to teach Qi Gong and use it for yourself, and your own health and wellbeing in all areas of life.

- **Liberty Forrest, Inspiring Speaker and Award-Winning Author Compassionate, Heart-Centered Guidance** libertyforrest.com

LIVE ONLINE COURSES

PurelandQiGong.com

Instructors Program
Remote Fa Chi Healing Program
Learn to Send Chi to the Needles
Using Chi to Heal Your Pets

Chi Gong: The Menopause Solution
Peri-menopause and post -menopause
ChangeTheEnergyKeepTheChange.com

CONTACT INFORMATION

Pureland International Qi Gong ™

http://www.PurelandQiGong.com

Social Media

http://www.instagram.com/PurelandQigong

https://www.youtube.com/c/PurelandQiGong

https://www.facebook.com/Qibreaks/ (one minute Qi Gong)

https://www.facebook.com/groups/QiGongGong

https://www.facebook.com/purelandqigong/

https://twitter.com/MasterTeresa

Meetup

https://www.meetup.com/eastmeetswestlightworkers/

https://www.meetup.com/Purelandqigong/

https://www.meetup.com/spiritual-community-usa/

Address

Teresa Yeung
Pureland International Qi Gong
355-8171 Yonge Street
Thornhill (Toronto North), Ontario Canada, L3T 2C6

Written by Teresa W. Yeung (Master Teresa®) with contributions by her students of Qi Gong

Book Editing by Sherree Felstead
http://www.passiontopaperpublishing.com

Cover Design by Rebecca Chan
http://www.rebeccachan.ca

ABOUT THE AUTHOR

It is extremely rare that a female becomes the successor of her master's Chi Gong lineage. Throughout the ages, blessings and teachings of the master are passed on to a worthy male student. Master Teresa Yeung is the sole successor to Grandmaster Weizhao Wu's Medical Qi Gong lineage, which he bestowed upon her before his passing to the spirit world in 2006. Grandmaster Wu was an educator and creator of the highly successful Wu's Eye Qi Gong® that has helped millions of people worldwide.

Master Teresa, while continuing to honor Grandmaster Wu's Qi Gong, has expanded the teachings to include balancing emotions, clearing limited beliefs, training healers; helping professionals and therapists integrate Qi Gong into their work. She is the founder of four registered private schools that specializes in different forms of Qi Gong and spread coast to coast:

Pureland International Qi Gong™
The Seventh Happiness® School of Chi Gong
Wu & Yeung® Qi Gong Wellness Institute
Wu's Qi Gong & Tai Chi® Fitness Centre Inc.

Not only is Master Teresa a healer, workshop leader, speaker and mentor, she is also a three-time #1 international bestselling and award-winning author:

Life Force: The Miraculous Power of Qi Gong - #1 Amazon Bestseller
Unlocking Your Happiness Within - #1 Amazon Bestseller
Unlocking Your Happiness Within Workbook
The Handbook to Holistic Health H₃ - #1 Amazon Bestseller

She won the Grand Trophy of 3rd Annual EZway Golden Gala Award and the Health Professional Award of the Year among 112 nominees in 2022. She has been featured and interviewed on various media: eZWay TV Broadcast, ABC, CP24, Omni TV, Fairchild TV, Rogers TV, radio, podcasts and health magazines. She has taught internationally in universities, elementary and high schools, hospitals, wellness centers, nutritional schools, traditional medical schools and naturopathic colleges and non-profit organizations.

Teresa is very passionate about helping her students, and they are just as passionate about learning from her! They have tremendous respect for her knowledge and ability to gauge their health concerns. They often describe her as energizing, uplifting, happy and friendly, and her love for healing is the real deal!

Master Teresa and her family are living examples of the positive transformation that Qi Gong has had on their lives. All three of her children: Rebecca, Daniel and Jacqueline are successful in their own right, as Master Teresa herself is an internationally recognized Master. That is why she is excited about passing on her knowledge to others. Whether there is physical, emotional, mental or spiritual suffering, she can help to release it.

Her online programs make it possible to reach students around the world training remote healers. They are able to listen to her philosophy and practice her insightful teachings from the viewpoint of a woman. She is also instructing practitioners from coast to coast to serve the growing demand for organic energy healing through Pureland Qi Gong®.

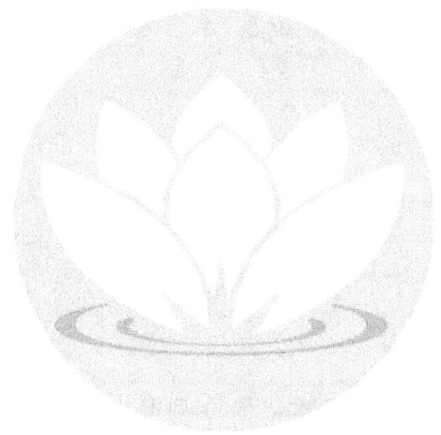

Pureland International Qi Gong

FIND YOUR CORE · FIND YOUR ROOTS · FIND YOUR PURPOSE